Prentice Hall Health

outline review

of Massage Therapy

Barbara B. Rice, BA, LMT
Lakeland, Florida

D1605495

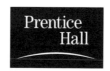

Prentice
Hall

Upper Saddle River, New Jersey 07458

Library of Congress Cataloging-in-Publication Data
Rice, Barbara B.
  Prentice Hall Health's outline review of massage therapy / Barbara B. Rice.
    p. ; cm. -- (Success across the boards) (Prentice Hall Health review series)
Includes bibliographical references and index.
  ISBN 0-13-048848-8
  1. Massage therapy--Outlines, syllabi, etc.
    [DNLM: 1. Massage--Outlines. WB 18.2 R495p 2002] I.
Title: Outline review of massage therapy. II. Title. III. Series.
IV. Series: Prentice Hall Health review series
  RM721 .R53 2002
  615.8'22'076--dc21

                                    2002009509

Notice: The author and the publisher of this volume have taken care that the information and technical recommendations contained herein are based on research and expert consultation, and are accurate and compatible with the standards generally accepted at the time of publication. Nevertheless, as new information becomes available, changes in clinical and technical practices become necessary. The reader is advised to carefully consult manufacturers' instructions and information material for all supplies and equipment before use, and to consult with a health care professional as necessary. This advice is especially important when using new supplies or equipment for clinical purposes. The author and publisher disclaim all responsibility for any liability, loss, or damage incurred as a consequence, directly or indirectly, of the use and application of any of the contents of this volume.

Publisher: Julie Levin Alexander
Assistant to Publisher: Regina Bruno
Acquisitions Editor: Mark Cohen
Assistant Editor: Melissa Kerian
Editorial Assistant: Mary Ellen Ruitenberg
Marketing Manager: Nicole Benson
Product Information Manager: Rachele Strober
Director of Production and Manufacturing:
  Bruce Johnson
Managing Production Editor: Patrick Walsh
Production Liaison: Alexander Ivchenko

Production Editor: Jessica Balch, Pine Tree Composition
Manufacturing Manager: Ilene Sanford
Manufacturing Buyer: Pat Brown
Design Director: Cheryl Asherman
Design Coordinator: Maria Guglielmo-Walsh
Cover and Interior Designer: Janice Bielawa
Composition: Pine Tree Composition
Manager of Media Production: Amy Peltier
New Media Project Manager: Stephen Hartner
Printing and Binding: Banta Book Group
Cover Printer: Phoenix Color

Pearson Education, Ltd., *London*
Pearson Education Australia Pty. Limited, *Sydney*
Pearson Education Singapore Pte. Ltd.
Pearson Education North Asia Ltd., *Hong Kong*
Pearson Education Canada, Ltd., *Toronto*
Pearson Educación de Mexico, S.A. de C.V.
Pearson Education—Japan, *Tokyo*
Pearson Education Malaysia, Pte. Ltd.
Pearson Education, Upper Saddle River, New Jersey

Dedicated to my parents RoseMarie Bartell Rice and John F. "Doc" Rice. Your example and intelligence has always been an inspiration to me. Thank you for allowing me into your world, for teaching me more than could ever be learned in books, and for always believing in me.

I would also like to thank the Sarasota School of Massage Therapy, especially Michelle Manna, who opened my heart and mind to the true gift of massage and giving.

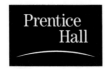

ISBN 0-13-048848-8

Contents

Preface

The National Certification Board for Therapeutic Massage and Bodywork (NCBTMB) examination is currently used in 23 states and numerous counties/townships as the sole examination for licensure as a massage therapist. For students of massage, preparing for this examination can be overwhelming. This review text is formatted as a concise and specific review of information on the NCBTMB and other state licensing exams, compiled through years of collecting questions from new student graduates, instructors and seasoned massage therapists who have sat for and successfully completed these examinations.

The subjects covered in this review book have been developed from the outline in the NCBTMB examination booklet. Information to be covered in the following four chapters will include: The Human Body, Anatomy and Pathophysiology, Muscle Movement and Anatomy, and Massage and the Business of Massage. At the end of each chapter, a 100-question examination is provided with rationale for each answer. A comprehensive 100-question examination is found at the end of the text and two additional 100-question examinations are on the CD-ROM that accompanies the text.

This manual contains the most current information in the field of massage therapy, and test questions parallel those that have been repeatedly asked over the last five years.

This publication will be the only review book necessary to successfully sit for and pass the NCBTMB examination.

Barbara B. Rice

Introduction

 ## SUCCESS ACROSS THE BOARDS:
THE PRENTICE HALL HEALTH REVIEW SERIES

Prentice Hall Health is pleased to present *Success Across the Boards,* our new review series. These authoritative texts give you expert help in preparing for certifying examinations. Each title in the series comes with its own technology package, including a CD-ROM and a Companion Website. You will find that this powerful combination of text and media provides you with expert help and guidance for achieving success across the boards.

COMPONENTS OF THE SERIES

The series is made up of a book and CD combination as well as a Companion Website that supports the book.

About the Book

Prentice Hall Health Outline Review of Massage Therapy **by Barbara B. Rice**

- *Study Questions:* The book has been designed to help the student prepare for the written certification exam. 400 multiple-choice questions are organized by all the topics covered on the exam and follow the exam format. Working through these questions will help you assess your strengths and weaknesses in each topic of study. Correct answers and comprehensive rationales are included. All questions are related to school textbooks so that you can quickly and easily find resources for more in-depth explanation or study on a specific topic.

- *Practice Exam:* An exam-like practice test with 100 questions is included at the end of the book. This test will give you a chance to experience the exam before you actually have to take it. These questions also include correct answers, comprehensive rationales, and references to the student text to assist you in determining your strengths, weaknesses, and needs for further study.

About the CD-ROM

A CD-ROM is included in the back of this book. The accompanying CD includes two 100-question examinations from material presented in the book. Correct answers and comprehensive rationales and references to the student text follow all questions. You will receive immediate feedback to identify your strengths and weaknesses in each topic covered.

Companion Website for Massage Therapy Review

Visit the website at *www.prenhall.com/review* for additional practice, information about the exam, and links to related resources. Designed as a supplement to this book in the series you will want to bookmark this site and return frequently for the most current information on your path to success.

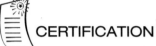

CERTIFICATION

The National Certification Board for Therapeutic Massage and Bodywork sponsors a national certification program for Massage Therapy. The components of the NCBTMB for massage therapy include:

1. Completion and documentation of a minimum of 500-hour training program from an accredited massage school.
2. Documentation of skills competency through the accredited massage school.
3. Passing a national written examination.

Since the program began in 1992, over 50,000 massage therapists have been certified through this national program which is legally recognized in 23 states, establishing a national standard for preparation of massage therapists. The names of all massage therapists who successfully complete all three components are placed in the national registry of certified massage therapists.

✓ ABOUT THE EXAM

The National Certification Examination is a computerized test administered by Assessment Systems, Inc., chosen by the NCBTMB. The exam is given throughout the United States at local test sites throughout the year. The examination contains 170 multiple-choice questions selected from the four major sections of required study in a massage therapy schools curriculum:

Section I (27%): Human Anatomy, Physiology and Kinesiology (Including Non-Western Studies)
Section II (20%): Clinical Pathology
Section III (41%): Massage Therapy and Bodywork: Theory, Assessment and Application
Section IV (12%): Professional Standards, Ethics and Business Practices

Information about the examination and an application may be obtained by contacting NCBTMB; 8201 Greensboro Drive, Suite 300, McLean, VA. 22102. 1-800-296-0664; *www.ncbtmb.com*

Information about the examination may change, so be sure to obtain current information by contacting NCBTMB.

STUDY TIPS

Review Materials

Choose review materials that contain the information you need to study. Save time by making sure that you aren't studying anything you don't need to. Before the exam, the best study preparation would be to use this Outline Review to identify your strengths and weaknesses. The references at the end of each rationale will direct you to additional resources for more in-depth study.

Set a Study Schedule

Use your time-management skills to set a schedule that will help you feel as prepared as you can be. Consider all the relevant factors—the materials you need to study, how many months, weeks, or days until the test date, and how much time you can study each day. If you establish your schedule ahead of time and write it in your date book, you will be much more likely to follow it.

Take Practice Tests

Practice as much as possible, using the questions in this book, on the accompanying CD, and the Web site. These questions were designed to follow the format of questions that appear on the exam you will take, so the more you practice with these questions, the better prepared you will be on test day.

The printed practice test in the back of the book and the practice tests on the CD will give you a chance to the experience the exam before you actually have to take it and will also let you know how you're doing and where you need to do better. For best results, we recommend you take a practice test 2 to 3 weeks before you are scheduled to take the actual exam. Spend the next weeks targeting those areas in which you performed poorly by reviewing questions in those areas.

Practice under test-like conditions—in a quiet room, with no books or notes to help you, and with a clock telling you when to stop. Try to come as close as you can to duplicating the actual test situation.

TAKING THE EXAMINATION

Prepare Physically

When taking the exam, you need to work efficiently under time pressure. If your body is tired or under stress, you might not think as clearly or perform as well as you usually do. If you can, avoid staying up all night. Get some sleep so that you can wake up rested and alert.

Eating right is also important. The best advice is to eat a light, well-balanced meal before a test. When time is short, grab a quick-energy snack such as a banana, orange juice, or a granola bar.

The Examination Site

The examination site should be located prior to the required examination time. It is wise to find the site and parking facilities the day before the test. Parking fee information should be obtained so that sufficient money can be taken along on the examination day.

Allow plenty of time for travel to the site in case of unexpected mishaps such as traffic snarls. During travel, think positive thoughts (e.g. "My preparation for the exam was thorough, so I'll be able to answer the questions easily"). Maintain a confident attitude to prevent unnecessary stress.

Materials

Be sure to take all required identification materials, registration forms, and any other items required by the testing organization or center. Read information and instructions supplied by the testing organizations thoroughly to be sure you have all necessary materials before the day of the exam.

Read Test Directions

Read the examination directions thoroughly! Because some board examinations have different test sections with different question formats, it is important to be aware of changes in directions. Read each set of directions completely before starting a new section of questions.

The examination is computerized. The computer is capable of keeping track of questions you have skipped, answered, and number remaining. Be sure to read and re-read each question before closing the program.

Selecting the Right Answer

Keep in mind that only one answer is correct. First read the stem of the question with each possible choice provided and eliminate choices that are obviously incorrect. Be cautious about choosing the first answer that might be correct; all possibilities should be considered before the final choice is made; the best answer should be selected.

If a question is complicated, try to break it down into small sections that are easy to understand. Pay special attention to qualifiers such as only, except, etc. For example, negative words in a question can confuse your understanding of what the question asks ("Which of the following is not…").

Intelligent Guessing

If you don't know the answer, eliminate those answers that you know or suspect are wrong. Your goal is to narrow down your choices. Here are some questions to ask yourself:

- Is the choice accurate in its own terms? If there's an error in the choice, for example, a term that is incorrectly defined—the answer is wrong.
- Is the choice relevant? An answer may be accurate, but it may not relate to the essence of the question.
- Are there any distractors, such as *always, never, all, none,* or *every*? Qualifiers make it easy to find an exception that makes a choice incorrect.

Mark answers you aren't sure of, and go back to them at the end of the test.

Ask yourself whether you would make the same guesses again. Chances are that you will leave your answers alone, but you may notice something that will make you change your mind—a qualifier that affects meaning or a remembered fact that will enable you to answer the question without guessing.

Watch the Clock

Keep track of how much time is left and how you are progressing. Wear a watch or bring a small clock with you to the test room. A wall clock may be broken, or there may be no clock at all.

Some students are so concerned about time that they rush through the exam and have time left over. In such situations, it's easy to leave early. The best approach, however, is to take your time. Stay until the end so that you can check your answers.

KEYS TO SUCCESS ACROSS THE BOARDS

- Study, Review, and Practice
- Keep a positive, confident attitude

- Follow all directions on the examination
- Do your best

Good luck!

You are encouraged to visit **http://www.prenhall.com/success** *for additional tips on studying, test-taking, and other keys to success. At this stage of your education and career you will find these tips helpful.*

1

The Human Body

contents

I. DIRECTIONAL TERMS

A. *Anatomical position*—body erect with palms facing forward; medical professionals always refer to the human body in the anatomical position.

B. *Abduction*—moving a body part away from the midline.

C. *Adduction*—moving a body part toward the midline.

D. *Bilateral*—on both sides.

E. *Cephalic/cranial/superior*—toward the head or upper part of the trunk.

F. *Caudal/inferior*—away from the head, toward the "tail," or lower than the point of reference.

G. *Centrifugal*—away from the center.

H. *Centripetal*—toward the center (all massage strokes are done centripetally).

I. *Circumduction*—circular movement of an extremity.

J. *Contralateral*—on the opposite side.

K. *Deep*—toward the core or away from the surface.

L. *Distal*—further away from the point of origin or point of reference; only used when referring to the limbs.

M. *Dorsal*—posterior or back of the body.

N. *Dorsiflexion*—moving the top of the foot and toes toward the head.

O. *Eversion*—soles of the feet directed away from each other.

P. *Extension*—creating more space between origin and insertion of a muscle.

Q. *Flexion*—creating less space between origin and insertion of a muscle.

R. *Inversion*—soles of the feet facing each other.

S. *Ipsilateral*—on the same side.

T. *Lateral*—away from the midline of the body or point of reference.

U. *Lateral flexion*—bending the neck so the ear goes to the shoulder; side bending.

V. *Medial*—toward the midline of the body or point of reference.

W. *Plantar-flexion*—pointing the toes away from the head.

X. *Pronation*—palms of hands facing posteriorly.

Y. *Proximal*—toward the trunk; closer to the point of origin or reference; only used when referring to the limbs.

Z. *Superficial*—toward the surface.

AA. *Supination*—palms of hands facing forward.

BB. *Unilateral*—on one side.

CC. *Ventral*—anterior or front of the body.

II. ORGANIZATION OF THE HUMAN BODY

A. Organization—All living organisms develop from the simplest to the most complex; the human body develops as follows: Atoms (H, O, K) to molecules (H_2O) to cells (basic structural and functional unit of an organism) to tissues (epithelial, muscle, connective, nervous) to organs (liver, stomach, heart) to organ systems (digestive, reproductive, circulatory) to organism (an individual)

1. Planes—divide the body into segments
    a) Coronal/frontal—divides the body into anterior and posterior halves
    b) Horizontal/transverse—divides the body into superior and inferior sections
    c) Midsagittal—divides the body into *equal* left and right halves
    d) Sagittal—divides the body into left and right sections
2. Cavities
    a) Dorsal
        (1) Cranial cavity (brain)
        (2) Vertebral cavity (spinal cord)
    b) Ventral
        (1) Thoracic (above the diaphragm; pleural cavities and mediastinum)
        (2) Abdominopelvic (below the diaphragm; digestive, excretory, and reproductive organs)
3. Abdominal quadrants

Upper Right (liver)	Upper Left (spleen, stomach)
Lower Right (appendix)	Lower Left (descending colon)

4. Abdominopelvic regions

Right Hypochondriac (liver)	Epigastric (liver, stomach)	Left Hypochondriac (left lobe of stomach)
Right Lumbar (ascending colon)	Umbilical (small intestine, transverse colon)	Left Lumbar (descending colon)
Right Iliac/Inguinal (cecum/appendix)	Hypogastric/Pubic (urinary bladder)	Left Iliac/Inguinal (descending colon)

2

Anatomy and Pathophysiology

contents

I. **HOMEOSTASIS**—the body working to maintain its internal environment; i.e., temperature regulation, urinary output, sweating

   A. **Metabolism**—the sum of two different types of chemical reactions within the body that work to maintain homeostasis
   1. Catabolism—the breakdown of complex molecules into simpler more usable atoms (generates energy)
   2. Anabolism—the building up of simple to complex (uses energy); i.e., anabolic steroids
      a) ATP—adenosine triphosphate (energy molecule within the body)

II. **THE CELL**

   A. **The cell is composed of *organelles* that serve a specific function**
   1. *Cell membrane*—keeps the cell whole; allows passage of material in and out of the cell
   2. *Cytoplasm*—fluid within the cell but outside the nucleus
   3. *Endoplasmic reticulum*—prepares protein for use in the cell and/or transport out of the cell
      a) Smooth—produce lipids
      b) Rough—produce protein; works with the golgi apparatus
   4. *Enzymes*—proteins
   5. *Golgi apparatus (complex)*—helps transport proteins and lipids to the plasma membrane, forms lysosomes and secretory vessels
   6. *Lysosomes*—digest material within the cell
   7. *Mitochondria*—"powerhouse" of the cell; generates ATP
   8. *Nucleus*—contains DNA; controls all cell activity
   9. *Ribosomes*—assemble proteins

III. **TRANSPORT SYSTEMS**

   A. **Active—*pinocytosis,* or cell "drinking"; *phagocytosis* or cell "eating"**

   B. **Passive—*osmosis,* diffusion of water from a higher concentration to a lower concentration gradient; *filtration*, water and dissolved particles from higher concentration to lower concentration (e.g., coffee maker); *diffusion*, substance movement from higher to lower concentration (e.g., aromatherapy)**

IV. **HISTOLOGY—THE STUDY OF TISSUES**

   A. **Tissues—made up of like cells that work together to perform a specific function**
   1. Connective tissue (vascular)—most abundant tissue in the body; it is responsible for binding structures together, connecting structures, and giving shape
      a) Areolar—most abundant; connects skin to underlying structures
      b) Adipose (fat)—insulates and stores energy

      c) Reticular—provides the framework for certain organs

      d) Cartilage—support, protection (nose, ears)

      e) Fibrous—tendons and ligaments

      f) Bone (osseous), blood (vascular)

2. Epithelial tissue (avascular)—lines organs, covers the body, forms glands

      a) Covering and lining—skin, inner and outer layer of organs; exposed to the outside (esophagus); functions include protection, secretion, excretion and absorption

      b) Glandular

        (1) Endocrine glands—secrete hormones directly into the blood

        (2) Exocrine glands—secrete hormones onto a free surface (skin) or into a duct; sweat glands

3. Muscle tissue—responsible for contracting muscles

      a) Skeletal—voluntary; attached to bone or other muscles; responsible for movement

      b) Smooth—involuntary; contraction of blood vessels, intestines

      c) Cardiac—involuntary; pushes blood from heart to blood vessels

4. Nervous tissue—controls all body functions by nerve impulses; consists of neurons (nerve cell) and neuroglia (supportive tissue)

B. Membranes

1. Epithelial—contain an epithelial layer and a connective tissue layer

      a) Mucous—line cavities that open directly to the outside of the body; keep respiratory and digestive tracts moist, fight bacteria, and secrete digestive enzymes

      b) Serous—keep organs and their cavities moist

        (1) Parietal—cavity wall

        (2) Visceral—covers and attaches organs to their cavities

        (3) Pleural—thoracic and lungs

        (4) Pericardium—heart and covering

        (5) Peritoneum—abdominal/pelvic

2. Synovial—line freely moveable joints; synovial fluid lubricates cartilage

      a) Bursae—sac or pouch of synovial fluid located at joints

      b) Tendon sheaths—cover the hands and feet

3. Fibrous connective tissue (fascial)

      a) Superficial—connects skin to underlying structures

      b) Deep—separates and connects muscle groups to bones

V. THE INTEGUMENTARY SYSTEM

A. Anatomy and physiology

1. Consists of the skin and its derivatives (hair, nails, nerve endings, glands)

2. The skin is considered an organ; its functions include temperature regulation (sweating), protection of internal structures, sensation

(heat, cold, touch), excretion (sweating, oil production), immunity (keeps bacteria from getting into the inner body), and synthesis of vitamin D (UV ray absorption)

3. Layers
   a) Epidermis—superficial layer; comprised of four or five layers; from superficial to deep
      (1) Layers of the epidermis
         (a) Stratum corneum—continually sheds
         (b) Stratum lucidum—only in hands and feet
         (c) Stratum granulosum—keratin is produced
         (d) Stratum basale (germinativum)—constantly dividing
      (2) Cells of the epidermis
         (a) Melanocytes—produce melanin, which absorbs UV light and is responsible for skin color
         (b) Merkle—sensation of touch
         (c) Langerhans—immunity; easily damaged by UV light
         (d) Keratinocytes—produce keratin, the waterproofing agent of the body
   b) Dermis—composed of connective tissue; thicker in soles of feet and palms of hands
      (1) Papillary region—tactile region; dermal papillae—fingerprints
      (2) Reticular layer—hair follicles, nerves, glands and fat; attaches to underlying structures by the hypodermis (superficial fascia)
      (3) Cells of the dermis
         (a) Fibroblasts—produce fibrin, which is responsible for blood clotting
         (b) Adipocytes—fat cells for cushioning and protection
         (c) Macrophage—part of the immune system

4. Glands
   a) Sebaceous—oil glands connected to hair follicles that produce sebum
   b) Sudoriferous—sweat glands
      (1) Eccrine—all over the skin but most numerous on palms and soles
      (2) Apocrine—armpit, pubic area
      (3) Ceruminous—found in the ear and produces cerumen (ear wax)

B. Aging—once we hit our late 40s, we experience significant changes in the structure and function of the skin; we begin to show wrinkles, our hair and nails grow slower, our immune system slows down, our skin becomes dry and fragile, sweat production slows, and there is a decrease in the amount of functional melanocytes (therefore we get gray hair and liver spots)

C. **Pathology of the integumentary system—fungal infections are highly contagious; if during the massage you come in contact with the infection, stop the massage; immediately wash your hands and avoid the area**

1. Burns—rated as 1st, 2nd, and 3rd degree; 3rd degree is the worst
2. Skin cancer—know the ABCDs (asymmetry, border, color, and diameter); always report suspicious looking moles to your client so he or she can alert a physician for further investigation
   a) Basal cell carcinoma—most common
   b) Squamous cell carcinoma—more severe
   c) Malignant melanoma—life-threatening
3. Fibrosis—scar tissue
4. Keloid scar—from original wound to surrounding tissue
5. Acne—involves an oil gland (massage is locally contraindicated)
6. Contusion—bruise; massage is okay in the yellow stage; ask client if there is any other pain associated with the bruise—same goes for hematomas (massage is locally contraindicated)
7. Cyst—fluid-filled sac; do not massage unless indicated by physician
8. Impetigo—bacteria/highly contagious; do not massage
9. Laceration—irregular tear of the skin (massage is locally contraindicated)
10. Nevus—birthmark
11. Pruritis—itching
12. Wart—virus (massage is locally contraindicated)
13. Furuncle—boil (massage is locally contraindicated)
14. Carbuncle—cluster of furuncles (massage is locally contraindicated)
15. Cellulitis—painful inflammation of underlying tissues; massage should be light
16. Keratoma—callus
17. Seborrhea—overactive oil glands (massage is locally contraindicated)
18. Rosacea—inflammation; overactive oil glands on cheeks and nose (massage is locally contraindicated)
19. Eczema—inflammation of the skin (massage is locally contraindicated)
20. Psoriasis—chronic, inflammatory; commonly concentrated on elbows, knees, chest, and scalp; not contagious, but area should be avoided because your lubricant and/or friction may aggravate the area
21. Dermatitis—inflammation of the skin
22. Tinea pedis—athlete's foot (fungal infection)
23. Tinea cruris—jock itch (fungal infection)
24. Tinea coporis—ringworm (fungal infection)
25. Ricket's disease—deficiency in vitamin D synthesis

D. **The most common benefits of massage on the integumentary system**
1. Stimulation of sensory receptors
2. Exfoliation
3. Moisturizing
4. Improved circulation
5. Increases perspiration (therefore opens up sweat/oil glands)
6. Overall enhancement of skin texture

VI. THE SKELETAL SYSTEM

A. **Anatomy and physiology**
1. Functions—support, protection, and movement, cell production, energy storage, and mineral storage
2. Bone—root word is *osseous;* prefix is *osteo-*
3. Cells—*osteoblasts* form bone; *osteocytes* maintain bone; and *osteoclasts* break down bone
4. *Spongy bone*—produces red blood cells (RBCs); where red bone marrow is found
5. *Hemopoiesis*—blood cell formation
6. Structure
   a) Long bone—longer than it is wide (femur, tibia, fibula, humerus, ulna, radius, and phalanges); *compact bone* (outer part of long bone) is composed of:
      (1) Diaphysis—shaft of the long bone
      (2) Epiphysis—ends of the long bone
      (3) Metaphysis—where the diaphysis and epiphysis meet
      (4) Articular cartilage—lines articulating (touching) surfaces of the epiphysis
      (5) Periosteum—where ligaments and tendons attach; covers the bone not covered by articular cartilage
      (6) Medullary cavity—contains yellow marrow (energy storage made up of adipose cells) in the diaphysis
      (7) Endosteum—lines the medullary cavity; contains osteoblasts and osteoclasts
   b) Short bones—carpals and tarsals
   c) Flat bones—ribs, sternum, frontalis, parietal, scapula
   d) Irregular bones—vertebrae
   e) Sesamoid bones—patella
7. Divisions—the human skeleton is divided into two categories:
   a) Axial—skull, hyoid, ribs, sternum and vertebrae
      (1) Skull (22 bones)
         (a) Cranial bones (8)—frontal (1), parietal (2), temporal (2), occipital (1), sphenoid (1), and ethmoid (1)
         (b) Facial bones (14)—nasal (2), lacrimal (2), zygomatic (cheeks, 2), inferior nasal concha (2), maxillary (upper jaw, 2), vomer (1), mandible (lower jaw, 1), palantine (palate, 2)

        (2) Hyoid—does not articulate with any other bone; serves as an attachment for muscles and supports the tongue

        (3) Ribs—12 pairs; 1–7 are true ribs, 8–12 are false ribs, and 11 and 12 are floating ribs

        (4) Sternum—manubrium (most superior), body (center), xiphoid process (most inferior) and an *endangerment site;* attachment site for the ribs and helps to protect the heart

        (5) Vertebrae—7 cervical (1st—atlas, 2nd—axis) (C1–C7), 12 thoracic (articulate with the ribs) (T1–T12), 5 lumbar (L1–L5), 5 sacral, 4 coccyx

   b) Appendicular—upper and lower extremities and their girdles

        (1) Pectoral (shoulder) girdle—clavicle (2), and scapula (2)

           (a) Acromioclavicular joint—where the acromion process articulates with the clavicle; the lateral joint

           (b) Sternoclavicular joint—where the sternum articulates with the clavicle; the medial joint

        (2) Upper limbs—humerus (2), ulna (2), radius (2), carpals (16), metacarpals (10), and phalanges (28)

           (a) Olecranon process—ulna; elbow

           (b) Colle's fracture—distal end of the radius is pushed back posteriorly

        (3) Pelvic (hip) girdle—hip, and pelvic bone

           (a) Hipbones consist of the ilium, ischium, and the pubis; together, they are called coxal bones

           (b) Pelvic girdle, sacrum, and coccyx form the pelvis

        (4) Lower limbs—femur (2), fibula (2), tibia (2), patella (2), tarsals (14), metatarsals (10), and phalanges (28)

           (a) Distal end of the tibia—medial malleolus; medial ankle

           (b) Distal end of fibula—lateral malleolus; lateral ankle

           (c) Pott's fracture—distal end of fibula breaks; serious injury results to the distal tibial articulation

B. Pathology of the skeletal system

1. *Osteoporosis*—decrease in bone density; kyphotic hump; massage with caution; no heavy pressure on the back or over joints; may be prevented or reversed with hormonal therapy, weight-bearing exercise, and diet

2. *Paget's disease*—excessive bone growth to replace extensive bone loss

3. *Osteoarthritis*—inflammation and pain associated with degeneration of articular cartilage; caused by overuse, injury, and weight placed on a joint

4. *Gout*—uric acid build-up; inflammation of big toe, extremely painful

5. *Herniated disc*—rupture of the fluid between the vertebrae, causing pressure posteriorly into a vertebral body; massage with physician approval

6. *Scoliosis*—abnormal lateral curvature of the spine through the sagittal plane
7. *Kyphosis*—"hump back," "dowager's hump"; exaggeration of the thoracic curvature
8. *Lordosis*—"sway back"; exaggeration of the lumbar curve

C. Articulations (joints—arthro)

1. Classifications—there are two classifications for joints
   a) Functional—identified by the space between the articulating bones
      (1) *Synarthrosis*—immovable joint
      (2) *Amphiarthrosis*—slightly moveable joint
      (3) *Diarthrosis*—freely moveable joint
   b) Structural—identified by their components
      (1) *Fibrous*—no synovial cavity; held together by connective tissue; a synarthrotic joint
         (a) Sutures—between cranial bones; gomphoses—between teeth and their sockets
         (b) Synchondrosis—epiphyseal plate
      (2) *Cartilaginous*—no synovial cavity; bones are joined together by cartilage; these joints are amphiarthrotic
         (a) Syndesmosis—between distal end of tibia and fibula
         (b) Symphysis—intervertebral discs and the pubic symphysis
      (3) *Synovial*—has a synovial cavity; diarthrotic
         (a) Gliding—tarsals and carpals
         (b) Hinge—elbow, knee, ankle, interphalangeal
         (c) Pivot—proximal radioulnar, atlantoaxial
         (d) Condyloid—radius and carpals, metacarpalphalangeal
         (e) Saddle—carpometacarpal joint of the thumb
         (f) Ball and socket—shoulder and hip
2. Pathology of articulations
   a) *Bursitis*—inflammation of the bursae; massage in the sub-acute stage, apply ice
   b) *Rheumatoid arthritis*—autoimmune disease; crippling and painful; massage in the sub-acute stage
   c) *Ankylosing spondylitis*—idiopathic (unknown cause); degenerative joint disorder; massage is indicated with caution
   d) *Sprain*—injury to the ligaments; 1st, 2nd, 3rd degree; massage in the sub-acute stage
   e) *Subluxation*—partial or incomplete dislocation; commonly treated by a chiropractor; physician indicates massage after treatment

D. The most common benefits of massage on the skeletal/articular systems

1. Improved joint mobility
2. Improved joint flexibility

3. Benefits are achieved through the therapist utilizing ROM exercises (active, passive, assisted), stretch/relax techniques (MET), and friction to tendons and ligaments

4. Massage should not be performed on a broken bone/area unless it is in the sub-acute stage where full bony union has been accomplished

VII. THE MUSCULAR SYSTEM

A. Anatomy and physiology

1. Tissues
   a) Skeletal (striated/voluntary)—attaches to bone and therefore moves parts of the skeleton
   b) Cardiac (striated/involuntary)—forms most of the heart
   c) Smooth (non-striated/involuntary)—blood vessels, stomach, and intestines

2. Functions of muscle tissue—motion, movements, maintaining posture, and generating heat

3. Characteristics of muscle tissue: excitability/irritability (ability to respond to stimuli), conductivity (ability to transmit stimuli), contractility (ability to shorten), extensibility (ability to stretch without injury), elasticity (ability to return to normal resting position/ shape after flexion)
   a) A muscle is strongest at its resting length
   b) *Flaccid*—muscle tone is diminished leaving the muscle to appear flat and loose
   c) *Atrophy*—wasting away of muscle from inactivity/non-use

4. Contraction of skeletal muscle—a motor unit receives an impulse from the brain/spinal cord, which stimulates the motor neuron to release acetylcholine; the acetylcholine stimulates the muscle fiber membrane, which stimulates the muscle fiber through the sarcoplasmic reticulum, to release calcium, which causes the actin and myosin to bind together and shorten the fiber, which contracts the muscle; ATP is used
   a) A motor unit consists of a neuron and all the cells it innervates
   b) Motor units respond in an all-or-none fashion to an action potential
   c) *Latent period* of a contraction is the time between the initial stimulus and when shortening begins; the *contraction period* is second and characterized by when the muscle contracts; the third is the *relaxation period,* where the muscle relaxes; the *refractory period* is when the muscle will not respond to a second stimulus because the first stimulus was strong enough to elicit a contraction
   d) *Fatigue*—muscles' inability to respond to stimuli because of oxygen depletion or waste build-up

5. Types of contractions
   a) *Isometric*—muscle length does not change, tension increases; an example is pushing your arms against a door jam

       b) *Isotonic*—muscle length changes, tension remains the same

         (1) Concentric—reduce the angle of a joint

         (2) Eccentric—length of muscle increases

       c) *Twitch*—brief contraction of all muscle fibers in a motor unit from a single action potential

       d) *Contracture*—inability of a muscle to relax after contraction

       e) *Tremor*—involuntary contraction of opposing muscle groups

       f) *Tetanus*—relaxation of a muscle is partial or not at all

       g) *Spasm*—involuntary contraction of a muscle/muscle group

       h) *Treppe*—repeated stimulation produces a contraction that is a little stronger than the first

       i) *Tic*—involuntary twitch that is usually controlled by voluntary muscles

   6. Connective tissue—continuous throughout the body and functions to surround and connect

       a) Tendons—connect muscle to bone

       b) Ligament—connect bone to bone

       c) Aponeurosis—sheet of connective tissue

       d) Chondrocytes are responsible for the maintenance of cartilage

         (1) *Superficial connective tissue*—below the skin and covers all of the muscular system

         (2) *Deep connective tissue*—surrounds muscle groups

            (a) Epimysium—surrounds individual muscles

            (b) Perimysium—surrounds muscle fibers (fascicles)

            (c) Endomysium—surrounds each muscle fiber

B. Pathology of the muscular system

   1. *Myasthenia gravis*—autoimmune disorder; weakness of skeletal muscles due to antibodies working against the acetylcholine receptor at the neuromuscular junction

   2. *Muscular dystrophy*—atrophy of skeletal muscle caused by degeneration of muscle fibers

   3. *Fibromyalgia*—painful condition with related "tender spots," stiffness of muscles and tendons; massage is indicated but MT should consult with physician

   4. *Lumbago*—pain in the lumbar region

   5. *Torticollis*—"wry neck" involves the SCM

   6. *Shin splints*—involve the periosteum around the tibia; treat with RICE (rest, ice, compression, elevation) and massage in the subacute stage

C. The most common benefits of massage on the muscular system

   1. Relief of muscular pain/discomfort

   2. Release of metabolic waste in muscle tissue

   3. Relaxation of muscle

   4. Improved muscular functioning

   5. Relief of muscle spasms

6. Improved tone and elasticity of muscle
7. Stimulation of cell activity, nerve supply, and circulation to muscle
8. Relieves stiffness and soreness
9. Improves rehabilitation rate of muscle injury
10. Friction prevents/reduces adhesion development after injury
11. ROM exercises will improve joint mobility and flexibility
12. Improved athletic performance
13. Prevent/alleviate delayed muscle soreness
14. Eliminate TP activity

VIII. THE NERVOUS SYSTEM

A. Anatomy and physiology—*neurology* is the study of the nervous system and disorders of the nervous system; the nervous system is the most complex system in the human body; it regulates all activities

1. The central nervous system consists of the brain and spinal cord
2. The peripheral nervous system
   a) Cranial nerves—brain (12 paired)
      (1) Cranial nerve X (vagus)—damage will affect smooth muscle control, specifically the abdomen and thorax; regulates the diaphragm
      (2) Cranial nerve XI (accessory)—damage will affect swallowing and movement of the head and lifting the shoulders (SCM and trapezius)
      (3) Cranial nerve VII (facial)—innervates the frontalis muscle
   b) Spinal nerves—spinal column (31 paired)
      (1) Sensory/afferent—send messages from sensory receptors to the CNS
      (2) Motor/efferent—send messages from CNS to muscles and glands
         (a) Somatic (voluntary)—control skeletal muscles
         (b) Autonomic (involuntary)—controls cardiac and smooth muscle, and glands
             i) Sympathetic—fight-or-flight; uses energy
             ii) Parasympathetic—regulates and conserves energy
         (c) Reflex—stimulus → sensory nerve fiber (impulse) → spinal cord → motor neuron → reflex
         (d) Reflex arc—pathway for a reflex
3. Nervous tissue
   a) Neurons (functional unit that carries impulses)—consist of axon (sends information away from cell body), cell body (nucleus, cytoplasm), and dendrites (input information to cell body)
      (1) A nerve is a bundle of nerve fibers (axons or dendrites) that extend from the CNS to the tissue that the neurons enervates
      (2) Neurological pathway—route that an impulse travels

(3) Myelin sheath—consists of lipids and proteins, and is found around axons; it insulates and helps to increase impulse conduction of a neuron

(4) An impulse leaves the axon, crosses the synapse where neurotransmitters carry the impulse to the dendrites through the cell body to the next axon terminals

b) Neuroglia (regulate the neurons)

4. Plexuses

a) Cervical plexus (C1–C5)—nerves that leave the vertebrae and affect the skin and muscles of the head, neck, and shoulder

b) Brachial plexus (C5–T1)—nerves that leave the vertebrae and affect the shoulder and upper limb; injury to the radial nerve results in the inability to extend the hand; median nerve damage causes inability to pronate the forearm and wrist flexion; ulnar nerve damage causes inability to adduct/abduct the fingers

c) Lumbar plexus (L1–L4)—nerves that leave the vertebrae and affect the abdominal wall, genitals and lower limb; femoral nerve damage causes inability to extend the leg

d) Sacral plexus (L4–S4)—nerves that leave the vertebrae and affect the buttocks, lower limbs; sciatic nerve damage causes pain radiating down the posterior leg

5. Sensory receptors

a) *Proprioceptors*—detect position and rate of movement

(1) Muscle spindle cells—located in the belly of the muscle; monitors length, stretch, and how far and fast a muscle is moving

(2) Golgi tendon organs—located in the tendon; monitor tension, stretching, and contracting

b) *Exteroceptors*—found close to the skin surface and relay information regarding the external environment (vision, smell, etc.)

c) *Visceroceptors*—information about internal organs

d) *Nociceptors*—pain receptors

e) *Thermoreceptors*—detect temperature changes

f) *Chemoreceptors*—detect chemical changes

g) *Photoreceptors*—detect light changes; located in the eyes

6. The brain

a) Brain stem—consists of three regions

(1) Medulla oblongata—regulates breathing, heartbeat, swallowing, and the blood vessels

(2) Pons—connects the spinal cord and brain; regulates respiration

(3) Mid-brain—regulates auditory and visual senses

(4) The brain stem also houses the limbic system, which regulates emotions

b) Cerebellum—regulates balance and voluntary movement

c) Diencephelon—houses the pineal gland

(1) Thalamus—detects pain, temperature, pressure, and cognition

(2) Hypothalamus—the "pleasure center"; regulates homeostasis

d) Cerebrum—speech, sensation, memory, reasoning; "the seat of intelligence"

B. Pathology of the nervous system

1. *Neuritis*—inflammation of a nerve
2. *Cerebral palsy*—loss of muscle control and coordination
3. *Parkinson's disease*—involuntary muscle movement interferes with voluntary
4. *Neuralgia*—pain along a peripheral sensory nerve
5. *Cerebrovascular accident* (CVA/stroke)—neurological deficits caused by blood clots or blood vessel hemorrhage; call 911 if one occurs during massage
6. *Transient ischemic attack* (TIA)—"mini-stroke"; temporary disruption of blood to the brain; call 911 if one occurs during massage
7. *Epilepsy*—short attack of motor, sensory or psychological dysfunction; it is okay to massage a client with a seizure disorder; if a seizure occurs during the massage, clear the area so your client will not hurt himself or herself; never hold the client down or attempt to place an object in his or her mouth

C. The most common benefits of massage on the nervous system

1. Interrupts noxious stimulation of pain
2. Stimulation through friction, percussion, and vibration massage
3. Relaxation through gentle effleurage and petrissage
4. Reflex effects on the internal organs, pain receptors, and muscles/joints
5. Stimulates parasympathetic activity (relaxation, endorphin release)
6. Increases body awareness through touch
7. Remember—all soft tissue is controlled by the nervous system

IX. THE ENDOCRINE SYSTEM

A. Anatomy and physiology

1. Pituitary—"master gland"; controlled by the hypothalamus

a) Anterior pituitary

(1) GH—growth hormone

(2) Prolactin—milk production after birth

(3) TSH—thyroid stimulating hormone; controls hormone secretions from the thyroid

(4) Adrenocorticotropic (ACTH)—stimulates adrenal cortex to secrete hormones

(5) Follicle stimulating hormone (FSH)—production of sperm in the testes and stimulating of follicles in ovaries

           (6) Leutinizing hormone (LH)—egg release in females and testosterone release in males

           (7) Melanocyte stimulating hormone (MSH)—stimulates release of melanin

      b) Posterior pituitary

           (1) Antidiuretic hormone (ADH)—regulates kidneys; decreases excretion of water

           (2) Oxytoxin—regulates uterus and mammary glands. Induces and controls contractions

2. Thyroid—neck (removes iodine)

    a) Thyroid hormones (T3/T4)—stimulates metabolism in body cells

    b) Thyroid stimulating hormone (TSH)—increases thyroid hormones (thyroxine)

    c) Calcitonin—decreases release of calcium from bones

      (1) *Hypothyroidism*—dwarfism

      (2) *Hyperthyroidism*—giantism

      (3) *Goiter*—enlarged thyroid gland; low levels of iodine in the body

3. Parathyroid gland—posterior surface of thyroid

    a) Parathyroid hormone (PTH)—regulates calcium; too much (hyper-) will result in high levels of calcium in the blood and will cause loss of calcium from bone; too little (hypo-) will interrupt normal functioning of muscle contractions

4. Adrenal glands—above the kidneys

    a) Epinephrine/norepinephrine—"fight-or-flight" response in the body; also called adrenaline/noradrenaline

    b) Aldosterone—involved with the sodium/potassium pump; decreases urine output by saving water

    c) Cortisol—metabolism, inflammation, and immunity

    d) Estrogen/testosterone—development of secondary sexual characteristics

5. Pineal gland—stimulated by light; responsible for the circadian (sleep/wake) cycles; releases melatonin

6. Pancreas—posterior to the stomach

    a) Exocrine function—secretes digestive enzymes into the duodenum

    b) Endocrine function

      (1) *Alpha cells* secrete glucagon when blood glucose levels are low

      (2) *Beta cells* secrete insulin when blood glucose levels are high

7. Thymus—behind sternum, and between lungs; increases white blood cell production

8. Ovaries/testes—estrogen and testosterone

9. Hormones only act on/affect specialized cells within the body (called target cells) by binding to receptors within those cells

B. Pathology of the endocrine system

   1. Diabetes mellitus

      a) *Type I*—deficiency in insulin; autoimmune; the body destroys its own beta cells; client is insulin dependent; insulin lowers blood glucose levels

      b) *Type II*—adult onset; 90% of all cases; over 40, overweight in typical client; too much insulin because target cells stopped working

   2. *Cushing's syndrome*—hypersecretion of cortisol; increases weight in abdomen; characteristic "moon face," "buffalo hump"; massage is indicated with physician referral

C. Benefit of massage on the endocrine system—massage will encourage the release of endorphins (natural painkillers)

X. THE CARDIOVASCULAR SYSTEM

A. Anatomy and physiology—the cardiovascular system consists of the heart, blood vessels, and blood

   1. Blood—transports, regulates, and protects; blood is created in bone marrow by a process called hemopoiesis; its components include:

      a) Blood plasma (55%)—water, dissolved proteins, ions, and urea

      b) Formed elements (45%)

         (1) Erythrocytes (RBCs)—live 120 days; bioconcave with no nucleus; carry hemoglobin (binds oxygen and carbon dioxide), nutrients, and oxygen

         (2) Leukocytes (WBCs)—live 1 week; granular or agranular; immunity

         (3) Thrombocytes (platelets)—clotting factor

   2. The heart

      a) Vagus nerve helps to control heart rate

      b) Layers of the heart from deep to superficial—endocardium, myocardium, epicardium

      c) Pulmonary circulation—blood flow to and from the lungs

      d) Coronary circulation—the heart has its own circulatory system; the body feeds the heart first

      e) Pericardium—encloses the heart

      f) *Sinoatrial node*—pacemaker; located in the R atrium

      g) *Atrioventricular valves*—between atrium and ventricles; left—bicuspid/mitral; right—tricuspid

      h) *Ventricular contraction*—1st sound in a blood pressure; systolic

      i) *Ventricular relaxation*—2nd sound in a blood pressure; diastolic

      j) Aorta branches—ascending (heart), brachiocephalic (head and arms), thoracic (chest), abdominal (abdominal contents), iliac (lower limbs)

      k) *Systole*—contraction of either the atria or ventricles in a complete cardiac cycle

      l) *Diastole*—relaxation of either the atria or ventricles in a complete cardiac cycle

3. Blood vessels
   a) Arteries and veins are named for where they are found
   b) Blood flows from the aorta → arteries → arterioles → capillaries → venules → veins
   c) Veins require skeletal muscular contraction and respiration to work effectively
   d) Great saphenous—longest vein in the body; from foot to femoral region; used in heart bypass surgery
   e) The center of a vessel where blood flows is called the lumen; an increase in the surface area is called *vasodilation;* a decrease in the surface area is called *vasoconstriction*
   f) *Pulse*—recoil of arteries after systole of the L ventricle
4. Systemic circulation (blood flow from the heart to the rest of the body)—*deoxygenated* blood flows into the R atrium → tricuspid valve → R ventricle → pulmonary semilunar valve → pulmonary trunk, which breaks into R and L pulmonary *arteries* where blood flows to the lungs and exchanges carbon dioxide for oxygen; *oxygenated* blood then flows from the lungs into the L and R pulmonary *veins* → L atrium → bicuspid valve → L ventricle → aortic semilunar valve → ascending aorta → systemic arteries → systemic capillaries where the exchange of oxygen and carbon dioxide takes place; all *deoxygenated* blood is then emptied into the superior vena cava (all blood superior to the heart), inferior vena cava (all blood inferior to the diaphragm), and coronary sinus (blood from the heart) and carried back into the R atrium

B. Pathology of the Cardiovascular System
1. *Anemia*—not enough working RBC or inability of RBC to carry oxygen
2. *Thrombosis*—formation of a clot (thrombus); once the clot breaks away it is called an embolus; if the embolus clogs a vessel and causes a decrease in blood flow it is called an embolism; an embolism in the heart will cause myocardial infarction (heart attack); in the brain it will cause a CVA (stroke); do not massage—you could release the thrombus
3. *Leukemia*—overproduction of leukocytes; leukocytes that won't die
4. *Raynaud's disease/syndrome*—vascular disorder in which the capillaries of the hands and feet are in spasm, restricting blood flow; typical discoloration from white to blue to red; pain, numbness, and tingling are associated with an attack; sufferers often complain of cold/numbness in feet and hands; can be brought on by cold or emotional stress; massage is indicated, but do not use ice
5. *Atherosclerosis*—plaque build-up
6. *Arteriosclerosis*—thickening of the walls of the arteries and loss of elasticity
7. *Arrhythmia*—irregular heartbeat
8. *Edema*—too much interstitial fluid, causing swelling

9. *Phlebitis*—inflammation of a vein
10. *Varicose veins*—enlarged veins can be caused by rupture or damaged valves
11. *Hypoxia*—lack of oxygen to the tissues
12. *Ischemia*—lack of blood flow to an area

C. **Massage and the cardiovascular system**
1. The most common benefits
   a) Improves/increases arterial circulation
   b) Improves/assists venous and lymphatic circulation
   c) May affect blood pressure and heart rate (lower)
   d) Produces hyperemia (influx of blood to an area) in the tissue
   e) Improves flow of interstitial fluid
   f) "Exercises" the blood vessels by manually constricting and allowing them to return to their normal size
2. Do not massage varicose veins; with deep pressure, the MT may dislodge a clot; same for phlebitis; if you are not sure, inform your client of your concern and contact client's physician before the next scheduled appointment
3. Massage for a client with hypertension (high blood pressure) should be light and soothing

XI. THE LYMPHATIC SYSTEM

A. **Anatomy and physiology**
1. Components—lymph, lymph organs, and lymph vessels
2. Function—immunity and transport; *antibodies*—proteins that attack invading organisms of the body; *antigens*—recognize foreign substances and attach to antibodies
3. Organs—red bone marrow, thymus gland (produces B and T cells), spleen (mass of lymph tissue, largest lymph organ, filled with blood not lymph, in L hypochondriac region)
4. How the lymphatic system works—lymph capillaries pick up fluid from the interstitial space and converge into lymph vessels (vessels are thinner and have more valves than veins; they are in the subcutaneous layer of the skin and follow veins) these vessels then converge to form lymph nodes (clustered in axilla, groin and mammary glands); fluid can get in but can't get out
   a) *Thoracic duct*—main lymphatic duct; goes into the L brachiocephalic vein

B. **Pathology of the lymphatic system**
1. *AIDS*—decrease in T4 cells
2. *Cancer*—immunity cells don't recognize that the cells are different and don't attack them; traditionally treated with drugs, radiation, and surgery
3. *Lymphoma*—lymphatic tissue tumor
4. *Lymphedema*—too much lymph causing edema
5. *Hodgkin's disease*—cancer usually arises in lymph nodes; idiopathic

6. *Chronic fatigue syndrome*—idiopathic; unexplained lethargy; massage is indicated with physician approval
7. *Lupus*—autoimmune, inflammatory disorder of connective tissue; symptoms include pain at the joints, fatigue/lethargy, photosensitivity, and a characteristic "butterfly rash" on the face; massage is indicated with physician approval
8. *Inflammation*—identified by redness, pain, heat, and swelling

C. The most common benefits of massage on the lymphatic system

1. Increases/improves the free flow of lymph
2. Assists lymph/waste into the proper channels for elimination
3. Lymphatic massage is always performed toward the nodes

XII. THE RESPIRATORY SYSTEM

A. Anatomy and physiology

1. Respiration
   a) *External respiration*—exchange of carbon dioxide and oxygen in the lungs
   b) *Internal respiration*—between systemic capillaries and cells
   c) *Cellular respiration*—within cells where chemical metabolism uses oxygen; gives off carbon dioxide and ATP is produced
2. The right lung contains three lobes and the left lung contains two lobes; this may help you to remember where the tricuspid and bicuspid valves are in the heart; the tricuspid valve is on the right side of the heart (three lobes in the lung) and the bicuspid valve is on the left side of the heart (two lobes in the left lung)
3. How we breathe—the diaphragm contracts (pushes downward), increasing space in the thoracic cavity, which draws air in through the nasal cavity and/or mouth; the air then passes through the larynx/pharynx to the trachea and into the bronchial tree, to the alveoli where gas exchange takes place (oxygen and carbon dioxide); the diaphragm relaxes (pushes up) and pushes air back out
   a) Tidal volume—the volume of one breath (complete inspiration and expiration)
   b) The pleural cavity/space contains a lubricant between the lungs and rib cage so that they can slide over each other when we breathe
4. Muscles associated with respiration
   a) Inspiration—diaphragm, external intercostals; forced inspiration—scalenes, SCM, serratus posterior superior, pectoralis minor
   b) Expiration—diaphragm, internal intercostals; forced expiration—all abdominals, internal intercostals

B. Pathology of the respiratory system

1. *Emphysema*—scar tissue replaces healthy tissue in the lungs
2. *Pulmonary embolism*—clot in the lungs; if it is a small clot it will cause dysfunction; a large clot will cause death

C. **The most common benefits of massage on the respiratory system**
   1. Through relaxation massage, respiration is decreased and deeper
   2. Tapotement to the thoracic region can help to break up respiratory congestion (phlegm)

XIII. THE DIGESTIVE SYSTEM

A. **Anatomy and physiology—the gastrointestinal (GI) tract (alimentary canal) is a tube that runs from the mouth to the anus; accessory organs of the digestive system: teeth, tongue, salivary glands, liver, gallbladder, and pancreas**
   1. Process of digestion—mouth (enzymes breakdown starch) → pharynx → esophagus → stomach (digestion of proteins, triglycerides, absorbs, coverts bolus to chyme [liquid]), → pyloric sphincter → small intestine: duodenum, jejunum, ilium (completes carbohydrate, protein, lipid and nucleic acid digestion) → ileocecal valve → large intestine: cecum, ascending, transverse, descending, sigmoid colons (the rest of water absorption and haustral churning takes place) → rectum → anus
      a) At the small intestine, the liver (bile for lipid digestion), gallbladder (stores bile) and pancreas (insulin) work to further break down and assist the chyme into the small intestine
      b) *Mastication*—chewing
      c) *Bolus*—ball of food
      d) *Mechanical digestion*—converting larger particles into smaller ones
      e) *Chemical digestion*—catabolic reaction
      f) *Peristalsis*—muscular contractions along the GI tract that push the food/bolus

B. **Pathology of the digestive system**
   1. *Cirrhosis*—scar tissue that develops in the liver from chronic inflammation; can be caused by alcoholism, hepatitis, or parasites; massage is indicated in the sub-acute stage; contact physician with any concerns
   2. *Hepatitis*—inflammation of the liver; can be caused by alcoholism, drugs, and viruses; massage is indicated in the sub-acute stage; contact physician with any concerns or if symptoms (jaundice, nausea, fever, chills) are present
      a) *Hepatitis A*—spread by fecal contact with food, utensils etc; contamination is commonly spread through inadequate handwashing after using the toilet
      b) *Hepatitis B*—spread through sexual contact, transfusions, dirty needles; can also be spread through saliva and tears
      c) *Hepatitis C*—spread through blood
   3. *Peritonitis*—inflammation of the peritoneum (serous membrane that encompasses the abdominal contents)

C. **The most common benefits of massage on the digestive system**
    1. Improves digestive processes through relaxation
    2. Abdominal massage will assist the movement of food by-products through the colon; always start in the descending colon and work to the ascending colon
    3. Abdominal massage can help regulate bowel movements

XIV. **THE EXCRETORY SYSTEM**

A. **Anatomy and physiology—the urinary system regulates blood pressure, water and electrolyte balance, and removes toxins**
    1. Components of the urinary system—kidneys, ureters, bladder, and urethra; the flow/route of excretion through the urinary system: kidneys → ureters → bladder → urethra
    2. Excretory organs
        a) Kidneys—eliminate uric acid, urea, electrolytes, and water
            (1) Nephron is the functional unit of the kidney
            (2) Renal refers to the kidneys
        b) Liver—forms urea, digestion of fats, conversion of amino acids into glucose or glucose into fatty acids, filters, neutralizes and detoxifies
        c) Large intestine—removes undigested material through defecation
        d) Lungs—remove carbon dioxide and water during exhalation

B. **Pathology of the excretory system**
    1. Cyst—prefix for words/pathology related to the bladder; i.e., cystitis—inflammation of the bladder; which may be characterized by the need to urinate frequently

C. **Benefit of massage on the excretory system—along with water intake, massage can help to eliminate toxins from the body**

XV. **THE REPRODUCTIVE SYSTEM**

A. **Anatomy and physiology**
    1. Male functions—production of hormones and sperm, copulation
        a) Testes are contained in the scrotum and produce testosterone and spermatozoa (contain DNA)
        b) Epididymis stores sperm until it is mature and moves into the vas deferens into the ejaculatory ducts and out the penis
        c) Semen—seminal fluid and sperm
        d) Seminal vesicles secrete seminal fluid into the ejaculatory ducts
        e) Prostate gland secretes a fluid to help the sperm move
        f) Cowper's gland produces mucus to lubricate the urethra
        g) Urethra carries urine or semen out of the body

2. Female functions—produce ovum (egg) and hormones, carries a fetus, copulation
   a) Vulva—external anatomy composed of labia major/minor
   b) Vagina—part of the birth canal
   c) Bartholen's gland—mucus producing glands
   d) Uterus—accommodates the fetus and fluids during pregnancy
   e) Fallopian tubes (oviducts)—propel the egg from ovaries; produce ovum, transport estrogen and progesterone to uterus
   f) Pregnancy—gestation
   g) Menopause—the cessation of menses; estrogen and progesterone decrease
3. Additional information
   a) A survivor of sexual abuse may exhibit inappropriate or what may appear as unusual responses during a massage; this may include sexual inappropriateness
   b) Clients who are diagnosed with dissociative disorder may exhibit unusual responses throughout the massage; it is important for the MT to constantly monitor clients and their responses, altering the massage to meet their changing needs

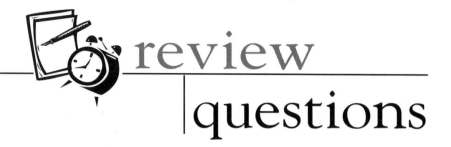

review questions

DIRECTIONS Each of the questions or incomplete statements below is followed by suggested answers or completions. Select the one answer that is best in each case.

1. Menopause causes what kind of hormonal changes?
   A. Increase in progesterone
   B. Increase in estrogen
   C. Decrease in estrogen
   D. Decrease in testosterone

2. Skin covering the soles of the feet is thicker because it consists of:
   A. More melanin.
   B. More keratin.
   C. More chondrocytes.
   D. Thicker dermis.

3. A client has a subluxation; to whom would you refer them?
   A. Chiropractor
   B. Podiatrist
   C. Respiratory therapist
   D. Urologist

4. A client reports having cystitis. What do you expect during the massage?
   A. Vomiting
   B. Need to urinate
   C. Cold hands
   D. Acne

5. An exaggerated curve through the sagittal plane is called:

   A. Lordosis.
   B. Kyphosis.
   C. Impetigo.
   D. Scoliosis.

6. Torticollis is also known as:
   A. Wry neck.
   B. Scoliosis.
   C. Ankylosing spondylitis.
   D. Slipped disc.

7. Which hormone is produced in the posterior pituitary?
   A. Aldosterone
   B. GH
   C. ADH
   D. FSH

8. A heart ventricle at rest after contraction is called:
   A. Systole.
   B. Diastole.
   C. Arrhythmia.
   D. Myocardial infarction.

9. The best treatment for bursitis is:
   A. Cold packs.
   B. Heat packs.
   C. Friction.
   D. Tapotement.

10. The ileocecal valve is located between the:
    A. Stomach and small intestine.
    B. Small intestine and large intestine.
    C. Esophagus and stomach.
    D. Gallbladder and liver.

11. Deficiency in lipid digestion is related to which organ?
    A. Spleen
    B. Small intestine
    C. Gallbladder
    D. Stomach

12. The best exercise to recommend to a client with osteoporosis is:
    A. Swimming.
    B. Weight lifting.
    C. Yoga.
    D. Stretching.

13. The golgi tendon is responsible for detecting change in muscle:
    A. Length.
    B. Striations.
    C. Composition.
    D. Tension.

14. The energy molecule of the body is:
    A. ACTH.
    B. ATP.
    C. GH.
    D. FSH.

15. Which of the following carries deoxygenated blood to the lungs?
    A. Pulmonary veins
    B. Pulmonary arteries
    C. Aorta
    D. Inferior vena cava

16. The fluid found in the pleural space:
    A. Makes the lungs more pliable.
    B. Makes the lungs expand.
    C. Provides lubricant between the lungs and rib cage.
    D. Provides blood to feed the alveoli.

17. The posterior pituitary gland regulates water absorption/excretion through the release of:
    A. Oxytoxin.
    B. Aldosterone.
    C. Prolactin.
    D. Antidiuretic hormone.

18. A client comes to your office and complains of being extremely emotional. Which system is responsible for the client's emotional state?
    A. Reproductive
    B. Limbic
    C. Circulatory
    D. Respiratory

19. Which muscle(s) are involved in forced expiration?
    A. External intercostals
    B. SCM
    C. Abdominals
    D. Scalenes

20. Gas exchange at the tissue/capillary level in the body is known as:
    A. Pulmonary respiration.
    B. External respiration.
    C. Internal respiration.
    D. Cellular respiration.

21. Which nerve innervates the frontalis muscle?
    A. Vagus (X)
    B. Facial (VII)
    C. Trigeminal (V)
    D. Trochlear (IV)

22. Lymphatic massage is performed:
    A. Away from the heart.
    B. Toward the nodes.
    C. Toward the feet.
    D. From prone to supine.

23. Indicators of gout include:
    A. Uric acid crystals/inflammation of the big toe.
    B. Headache/inflammation of the thumb.
    C. Astigmatism/rosacea.
    D. Color blindness/hearing loss.

24. In Western medicine, which is not a conventional treatment for cancer?
    A. Radiation
    B. Chemotherapy/drugs
    C. Physical therapy
    D. Surgery

25. Symptoms of Raynaud's disease include:
    A. Nosebleeds.
    B. Profuse sweating.
    C. Deformed joints.
    D. Discoloring/coldness of hands and feet.

26. Osteoporosis can be prevented or reversed by all of the following except:
    A. Hormone therapy.
    B. Exercise.
    C. Diet.
    D. Massage.

27. A client reports having epilepsy. During the massage, she has a seizure. What should you do?
    A. Put something in her mouth so she doesn't swallow her tongue.
    B. Put her into a seated position.
    C. Remove all objects around her so she doesn't get hurt.
    D. Hold her down on her back so she doesn't move around.

28. While massaging a client, a muscle contraction releases. What proprioceptor is involved?
    A. Spindle cells
    B. Golgi tendon
    C. Chemoreceptors
    D. Thermoreceptors

29. If a child is deficient in vitamin D, which disease can result?
    A. Scabies
    B. Scurvy
    C. Rickets
    D. Raynaud's

30. Contractility of a muscle is defined as the ability of a muscle to:

A. Return to its original shape after contraction.
B. Stretch.
C. Receive and react to stimuli.
D. Contract or shorten.

31. Which vitamin is emitted by the sun and absorbed through the skin?
    A. Vitamin A
    B. Vitamin D
    C. Vitamin K
    D. Vitamin E

32. Irritability of a muscle is defined as the ability of a muscle to:
    A. Return to its original shape after contraction.
    B. Stretch.
    C. Receive and react to stimuli.
    D. Contract or shorten.

33. An increase in the lumen of the vein is called:
    A. Vasoconstriction.
    B. Phlebitis.
    C. Vasodilation.
    D. Thrombosis.

34. Percussion over the thoracic region is best used to:
    A. Mobilize secretions.
    B. Test for broken ribs.
    C. Adjust a rib.
    D. Stretch the external intercostals.

35. Which pigmentation should you report to your client?
    A. Moles all over the body
    B. Moles with different color, shape, and size
    C. You do not report any suspicious moles because you don't want to scare your client.
    D. Moles are not something to worry about.

36. One complete cycle of inhalation and expiration is known as:
    A. Cellular respiration.
    B. Forced expiration.

C. Forced inspiration.

D. Tidal volume.

37. The spine and sternum protect the:
    A. Heart.
    B. Trachea.
    C. Kidneys.
    D. Liver.

38. Which bone is most superior to the ulna/radius?
    A. Femur
    B. Clavicle
    C. Talus
    D. Calcaneus

39. A client presents with variscosities in the leg. If you massage, what might occur?
    A. You will rid the leg of the variscosity.
    B. You will improve the tone of the veins.
    C. You will release a thrombus.
    D. You will see an instant change in the color of the feet.

40. A client presents with a bruise on the leg. What question should you ask before the massage?
    A. Do you have any other pain?
    B. Where did this occur?
    C. Have you put heat on it?
    D. Did you pinch yourself?

41. A client writes on the intake form that he suffers from rheumatoid arthritis. What symptoms should you expect?
    A. Uric acid build-up with inflamed big toe
    B. Red, white, and blue fingers and toes
    C. Bone growth in ear with loss of hearing
    D. Deformation of joint, pain and inflammation

42. Proprioceptors identify which of the following?
    A. Light changes in the environment and pupils
    B. Pain and directions of movement
    C. Position of body parts and directions of movement

D. Chemical changes and position of body parts

43. Kyphosis is defined as an exaggeration of the:
    A. Lumbar curvature of the spine.
    B. Thoracic curvature of the spine.
    C. Lateral curvature of the spine.
    D. Curvature of L1 to L4.

44. The correct medical nomenclature for "swayback" is:
    A. Scoliosis.
    B. Kyphosis.
    C. Lordosis.
    D. Ankylosing spondylitis.

45. Massage over varicose veins is:
    A. Encouraged.
    B. Done to eliminate the protrusion of the vein through the skin.
    C. Not advisable.
    D. Only done with legs elevated.

46. The direction of urine output is:
    A. Bladder, ureters, urethra, kidneys.
    B. Kidneys, urethra, ureters, bladder.
    C. Urethra, ureters, kidneys, bladder.
    D. Kidneys, ureters, bladder, urethra.

47. Diarthrotic joints are:
    A. Freely moveable.
    B. Slightly moveable.
    C. Sutures.
    D. Symphysis.

48. The "master gland" of the endocrine system is the:
    A. Thymus.
    B. Pituitary.
    C. Adrenal.
    D. Thyroid.

49. The nephron is the functional unit of the:
    A. Cell.
    B. Nervous system.
    C. Circulatory system.
    D. Kidney.

50. The pyloric sphincter is located between the:
    A. Small intestine and large intestine.
    B. Stomach and small intestine.
    C. Stomach and esophagus.
    D. Rectum and anus.

51. A motor neuron sends information from:
    A. CNS to muscles/glands.
    B. Sensory receptors to CNS.
    C. ANF to PNS.
    D. PNS to ANF.

52. Stimulation of the sympathetic nervous system will:
    A. Increase heart rate.
    B. Decrease heart rate.
    C. Decrease tidal volume.
    D. Increase insulin dependence.

53. Which vein is commonly used in heart bypass surgery?
    A. Femoral
    B. Subclavian
    C. Great saphenous
    D. Inferior vena cava

54. The small intestine is composed of (ascending to descending):
    A. Jejunum, ileum, duodenum.
    B. Ileum, duodenum, jejunum.
    C. Duodenum, ileum, jejunum.
    D. Duodenum, jejunum, ileum.

55. Which gland is responsible for the secretion of adrenaline?
    A. Thyroid
    B. Adrenal
    C. Thymus
    D. Pineal

56. Which valve is located between the right atrium and ventricle?
    A. Tricuspid
    B. Bicuspid
    C. Semilunar
    D. Mitral

57. Which of the following connects bone to bone?
    A. Tendon
    B. Ligament
    C. Linea aspera
    D. Styloid process

58. Which of the following is the most abundant tissue in the human body?
    A. Nervous
    B. Serous
    C. Epithelial
    D. Connective

59. The passage of food through the intestinal tract is possible because of:
    A. Mastication.
    B. Fermentation.
    C. Peristalsis.
    D. Defibrillation.

60. Which tissue lines cavities that open to the outside of the body?
    A. Epithelial
    B. Nervous
    C. Skeletal
    D. Connective

61. The pulmonary veins carry _____ blood from the lungs to the heart.
    A. Oxygenated
    B. Deoxygenated
    C. Carbon dioxide–rich
    D. Carbon monoxide–rich

62. Which of the following is not part of the axial skeleton?
    A. Hyoid
    B. Ribs
    C. Clavicle
    D. Vertebrae

63. From fine to gross, which is the order of connective tissue fascia that surrounds the muscles?
    A. Epimysium, endomysium, perimysium
    B. Endomysium, epimysium, perimysium

C. Perimysium, epimysium, endomysium
D. Endomysium, perimysium, epimysium

64. The "powerhouse" or energy organelle of a cell is the:
   A. Lysosome.
   B. Mitochondria.
   C. Golgi apparatus.
   D. Ribosome.

65. After a muscular contraction, a muscle loses the ability to respond to stimulation. This is known as the _____ period.
   A. Latent
   B. Refractory
   C. Relaxation
   D. Contraction

66. Chemical reactions where energy molecules are built-up are called:
   A. Ionic.
   B. Anabolic.
   C. Catabolic.
   D. Covalent.

67. The movement of water through a semi-permeable membrane is called:
   A. Diffusion.
   B. Active transport.
   C. Filtration.
   D. Osmosis.

68. Which of the following is where gas exchange takes place in the lungs?
   A. Bronchi
   B. Alveoli
   C. Pulmonary artery
   D. Pulmonary vein

69. The principle function of insulin is to:
   A. Lower blood glucose levels.
   B. Raise blood glucose levels.
   C. Lower CBC.
   D. Raise CBC.

70. The movement of molecules or ions from an area of higher concentration to an area of lower concentration is called:
   A. Osmosis.
   B. Diffusion.
   C. Filtration.
   D. Active transport.

71. The ingestion of a solid particle by a cell is called:
   A. Pinocytosis.
   B. Phagocytosis.
   C. Osmosis.
   D. Diffusion.

72. The part of the brain responsible for coordination and balance is called the:
   A. Cerebellum.
   B. Cerebrum.
   C. Medulla.
   D. Thalamus.

73. Which muscle fibers are striated and voluntary?
   A. Cardiac
   B. Skeletal
   C. Visceral
   D. Serous

74. The molecule that binds oxygen and carbon dioxide in erythrocytes is:
   A. Antigen.
   B. Thrombin.
   C. Hemoglobin.
   D. Globulin.

75. The waterproofing protein produced by cells of the epidermis is called:
   A. Antigen.
   B. Keratin.
   C. Melanin.
   D. Melatonin.

76. The basic structural and functional unit of all living things is the:
   A. Nephron.   C. Cell.
   B. Cytoplasm.   D. Tissue.

77. Sweat is produced by the:
    A. Sudoriferous glands.
    B. Sebaceous glands.
    C. Endocrine glands.
    D. Reproductive glands.

78. Which cells from the pancreas secrete insulin?
    A. Alpha cells
    B. T4 cells
    C. T3 cells
    D. Beta cells

79. The gland responsible for our sleep–wake cycle is called the:
    A. Thyroid.
    B. Pineal.
    C. Thymus.
    D. Pituitary.

80. The liver is located in the:
    A. Upper-right quadrant.
    B. Lower-right quadrant.
    C. Upper-left quadrant.
    D. Lower-left quadrant.

81. Which of the following cells are responsible for the maintenance of cartilage?
    A. Erythrocytes
    B. Leukocytes
    C. Thrombocytes
    D. Chondrocytes

82. The cells involved with the immune system are called:
    A. Erythrocytes.
    B. Leukocytes.
    C. Thrombocytes.
    D. Chondrocytes.

83. A muscle contraction in which the muscle fiber length is constant is called:
    A. Isotonic.
    B. Isometric.
    C. Concentric.
    D. Eccentric.

84. Which plane divides the body into anterior and posterior portions?
    A. Mid-sagittal.
    B. Sagittal.
    C. Transverse.
    D. Frontal.

85. Which type of gland secretes their hormones directly into the bloodstream?
    A. Exocrine
    B. Connective
    C. Endocrine
    D. Migratory

86. Which type of membrane provides a "slippery" surface area for organs and their cavities?
    A. Serous
    B. Cutaneous
    C. Synovial
    D. Mucous

87. Name the parts of the colon from the end of the small intestine to the rectum.
    A. Ileocecal valve, ascending colon, descending colon, transverse colon, sigmoid colon
    B. Ascending colon, iliocecal valve, transverse colon, sigmoid colon, descending colon
    C. Transverse colon, iliocecal valve, ascending colon, sigmoid colon, descending colon
    D. Ileocecal valve, ascending colon, transverse colon, descending colon, sigmoid colon

88. Haustral churning takes place in the:
    A. Stomach.
    B. Small intestine.
    C. Large intestine.
    D. Esophagus.

89. What should you do during a massage when you realize you have come in contact with a fungal infection?
    A. Stop massaging the area and continue on with the rest of the body.
    B. Stop the massage and wash your hands.

C. Don't worry because fungal infections are not contagious.

D. Ask the client if they would like you to wash the area.

90. The correct medical nomenclature for a heart attack is:
    A. Cerebrovascular accident.
    B. Transient ischemic attack.
    C. Myocardial infarction
    D. Hemiplasia.

91. Which joint exists only between the carpal and metacarpal bones of the thumb?
    A. Saddle.
    B. Hinge.
    C. Ellipsoidal.
    D. Gliding.

92. Excessive accumulation of fluid in the interstitial space is known as:
    A. Diastole.
    B. Edema.
    C. Hyperemia
    D. Ischemia.

93. A muscular contraction in which the length of the muscle shortens is called:
    A. Isometric.
    B. Static.
    C. Isotonic.
    D. Excentric.

94. While massaging someone with osteoporosis, the MT should be cautious of:
    A. Friction.
    B. Petrissage.
    C. Pressure on the back.
    D. None of the above.

95. A client reports having broken his ankle two weeks ago. You should:
    A. Proceed with the massage, healing has already begun.
    B. Proceed with the massage using deep transverse friction to ligaments and tendons.

C. Proceed with the massage doing range of motion to the ankle.

D. Proceed with the massage, avoiding the area until full bony union is accomplished.

96. The neurotransmitter released at the skeletal neuromuscular junction is called:
    A. ACH.
    B. GH.
    C. FSH.
    D. LH.

97. The aorta branches into which three trunks?
    A. Axillary, cranial, femoral
    B. Brachiocephalic, thoracic, abdominal
    C. Peroneal, cranial, abdominal
    D. Brachiocephalic, femoral, axillary

98. The lymph organ located in the upper-left quadrant is called:
    A. Liver.
    B. Stomach.
    C. Appendix.
    D. Spleen.

99. The connective tissue composed of cells specialized for fat storage is called:
    A. Blood.
    B. Loose.
    C. Adipose.
    D. Dense.

100. For muscular contraction to occur, which of the following molecules are needed?
    A. Actin, myosin
    B. Calcitonin, tropin
    C. Myosin, melanin
    D. Actin, tropin

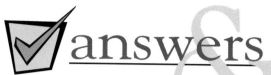
answers & rationales

The answer key will give you three pieces of information. The first is the correct answer, the second is the rationale, and the third is the section in the review book (or your own anatomy text) where you will find more information about the answer.

1.
C. Estrogen and progesterone decrease. (The Reproductive System)

2.
D. Keratin is the waterproofing agent. (The Integumentary System)

3.
A. Urologist—urology; physical therapist—soft tissue; podiatrist—foot. (The Skeletal System)

4.
B. Cyst–bladder. (The Excretory System)

5.
D. Key phrase: sagittal plane. (The Skeletal System)

6.
A. Think of a tortoise. (The Muscular System)

7.
C. Both B and D—anterior pituitary; A—kidneys. (The Endocrine System)

8.
B. Systole—contraction. (The Cardiovascular System)

9.
A. *Itis*—inflammation. Never apply heat to an inflamed area. (The Skeletal System)

10.
B. Ileum—small intestine; cecum—large intestine. (The Digestive System)

11.
B. Gallbladder—stores bile. (The Digestive System)

12.
B. Weightlifting will help to strengthen muscles and attachments. (The Skeletal System)

13.
D. Spindle cell detects changes in length and speed. (The Nervous System)

14.
B. The other choices are hormones. (The Human Body)

15.
B. The only arteries that carry deoxygenated blood. (The Cardiovascular System)

16.
C. Fluid found in cavities allows structures to glide over one another. (The Respiratory System)

17.
D. Diuretics increase the amount of urine output. Antidiuretics do the opposite. (The Endocrine System)

18.
B. This system is responsible for our emotional state. (The Nervous System)

19.
C. Internal intercostals are involved in forced expiration also. (The Respiratory System)

20.
C. Cellular respiration is within cells. (The Respiratory System)

21.
B. The facial (face). The frontalis muscle is part of the forehead. (The Nervous System)

22.
B. Lymphatic massage is always directed toward the lymph nodes. (The Lymphatic System)

23.
A. The most common complaint is pain in the big toe. (The Skeletal System)

24.
C. Physical therapy is not a traditional treatment for cancer. (The Lymphatic System)

25.
D. This is an impaired circulatory disorder. (The Cardiovascular System)

26.
D. Massage may help muscle tightness but cannot reverse it. (The Skeletal System)

27.
C. Never attempt to put anything in the mouth. (The Nervous System)

28.
A. Golgi tendon recognizes tension on the muscle. (The Nervous System)

29.
C. Scabies—bugs burrow in the skin; scurvy—vitamin C deficiency. (The Integumentary System)

30.
D. Contractility—contract. (The Muscular System)

31.
B. Deficiency will result in rickets. (The Integumentary System)

32.
C. Irritability—ability to be irritated by a stimulus. (The Muscular System)

33.
C. Vasoconstriction is a decrease in the diameter of the lumen. (The Cardiovascular System)

34.
A. B and C are beyond your scope of practice; D does not involve percussion. (The Respiratory System)

35.
B. Remember A, B, C, D—asymmetry, border, color, and diameter. (The Integumentary System)

36.
D. Cellular respiration—within the cell. (The Respiratory System)

37.
A. Anteriorly and posteriorly the heart is surrounded. (The Skeletal System)

38.
B. The other three choices are in the lower body. (The Skeletal System)

39.
C. Never massage over varicose veins. (The Cardiovascular System)

40.
A. You need to know if there are any other injuries. (The Integumentary System)

41.

D. A is gout; B is Raynaud's symptoms; C is Paget's symptoms. (The Skeletal System)

42.

C. A is photoreceptors, B is nociceptors, D is two different receptors. (The Nervous System)

43.

B. A is lordosis; C is scoliosis. (The Skeletal System)

44.

C. Kyphosis is also known as "hunchback." (The Skeletal System)

45.

C. Never massage over varicose veins; you may loosen a clot. (The Cardiovascular System)

46.

D. Key word: output. (The Excretory System)

47.

A. Amphiarthrotic—slightly moveable (symphysis); sutures are immovable. (The Skeletal System)

48.

B. Together with the hypothalamus, regulates almost all growth, development, and metabolism. (The Endocrine System)

49.

D. Nephros—kidney. (The Excretory System)

50.

B. Pylorus—part of the stomach. Pyle—gate. (The Digestive System)

51.

A. Motor neurons send information away from the CNS to produce movement. (The Nervous System)

52.

A. Sympathetic—fight or flight. (The Nervous System)

53.

C. Largest vein in the body. (The Cardiovascular System)

54.

D. Try to remember DJI. (The Digestive System)

55.

B. The answer is in the question—adrenaline (adrenal). (The Endocrine System)

56.

A. Remember three lobes in the right lung—tri. (The Cardiovascular System)

57.

B. Tendons connect muscle to bone. (The Muscular System)

58.

D. Surrounds and connects can be deep and superficial. (Histology)

59.

C. Mastication—chewing; fermentation—chemical process; defibrillation—procedure done for the heart. (The Digestive System)

60.

A. Can be moist to assist in excretion or act as a filter. (Histology)

61.

A. The only veins that carry oxygenated blood. (The Cardiovascular System)

62.

C. Axial—axis. The only choice not directly on the axis of the body. (The Skeletal System)

63.

D. Endo—within; peri—around; epi—upon. (The Muscular System)

64.

B. Think of "mighty." (Anatomy & Pathophysiology)

65.

B. Known as the period of lost excitability. (The Muscular System)

66.

B. Remember: Anabolic steroids build up muscle bulk. (Anatomy & Pathophysiology)

67.
D. Key word—water. (Anatomy & Pathophysiology)

68.
B. The only choice listed that resides in the lungs. (The Respiratory System)

69.
A. Glucagon raises blood glucose levels, insulin lowers it. (The Endocrine System)

70.
B. Think of diffusing essential oils. (Anatomy & Pathophysiology)

71.
B. Pinocytosis—cell drinking. (Anatomy & Pathophysiology)

72.
A. Cerebrum—"seat of intelligence." (The Nervous System)

73.
B. Key word—voluntary. (The Muscular System)

74.
C. Thrombin—involved in clot formation. (The Cardiovascular System)

75.
B. Melanin—coloring agent; melatonin—sleep/wake cycle. (The Integumentary System)

76.
C. Nephron—kidney; cytoplasm—within the cell; tissue—made up of cells. (The Human Body)

77.
A. Sebaceous—oil. (The Integumentary System)

78.
D. Alpha—secrete glucagon; T3/T4—stimulate metabolism. (The Endocrine System)

79.
B. Secretes melanin. (The Endocrine System)

80.
A. Upper left—stomach. (The Human Body)

81.
D. Chondros—cartilage. (The Muscular System)

82.
B. Erythrocytes—RBC. (The Cardiovascular System)

83.
B. Isometric—muscle length remains the same, tension increases. (The Muscular System)

84.
D. Mid-sagittal—equal R and L halves; sagittal—L and R sections; frontal—anterior and posterior portions. (The Human Body)

85.
C. Exocrine—secrete hormones onto a free surface or duct. (Anatomy & Pathophysiology)

86.
A. Key words—organs and their cavities. (Anatomy & Pathophysiology)

87.
D. The last component of the small intestine is the ileum. Then ascending, transverse, descending, and sigmoid colon in the large intestine. (The Digestive System)

88.
C. Key phrase—haustral churning. (The Digestive System)

89.
B. Fungal infections are contagious. (The Integumentary System)

90.
C. CVA—stroke, TIA—mini stroke; hemiplasia—term related to a stroke. (The Cardiovascular System)

91.
A. The only one in the body. (The Skeletal System)

92.
B. Hyperemia—excess of blood to an area; ischemia—lack of blood to an area. (The Cardiovascular System)

93.
C. Isotonic—tension remains the same, muscle length changes. (The Muscular System)

94.
C. Extreme pressure on the back may cause a fracture. (The Skeletal System)

95.
D. Do not massage a broken bone until the doctor reports that full bony union has been achieved. (The Skeletal System)

96.
A. The other three choices are hormones are responsible for growth and reproductive functions. (The Skeletal System)

97.
B. The three major trunks: brachio (arm) cephalic (head); thoracic—chest; abdominal—abdomen. (The Cardiovascular System)

98.
D. Key word—lymph organ. (The Human Body)

99.
C. Adipose—fat. (Anatomy & Pathophysiology)

100.
A. Tropins stimulate other endocrine glands; melanin is responsible for skin color. (The Muscular System)

3

Muscle Movement and Anatomy

contents

The majority of questions on licensing examinations are geared toward your knowledge of location and movement of a muscle rather than origin and insertion. A few questions may concern origin and insertion and bony landmarks (attachment sites of muscles), and it is assumed that you are familiar with this information. The questions in this section address all aspects of muscle movement/anatomy and require critical thinking regarding the movement of the human body.

In this section, the *agonist* (the muscle being referred to or the primary mover) is listed with *synergists* (muscles that perform the same movement as the *agonist*), and are listed in *order of strength* (the strongest muscle is listed first in a series). The *antagonists* (muscles that perform the opposite muscle function of the *agonist*) are identified in the text.

I. MUSCLES THAT MOVE THE HEAD

A. Flexors (bring the chin to the chest; antagonists to the extensors)
1. Sternocleidomastoid (bilaterally)
2. Scalenes

B. Extensors (bring the head backward; antagonists to the flexors)
1. Splenius capitis (bilaterally)
2. Splenius cervicis (bilaterally)

C. Rotation of head to same side
1. Splenius capitis (unilaterally)
2. Splenius cervicis (unilaterally)

D. Rotation of head to opposite side
1. Sternocleidomastoid (unilaterally)
2. Scalenes (unilaterally)

E. Lateral flexion (bring ear toward shoulder)
1. Sternocleidomastoid (unilaterally)
2. Scalenes (unilaterally)
3. Splenius capitis (unilaterally)
4. Splenius cervicis (unilaterally)

F. Helpful hints
1. Sternocleidomastoid (SCM) is named for its O & I; do not massage bilaterally because of the common carotid artery; it is an accessory muscle for breathing
2. SCM is the muscle responsible for torticollis (wry neck)
3. The scalenes also raise the ribs during forced inspiration (bilaterally)
4. The scalenes are known as an entrapper because it can entrap the brachial plexus; accessory muscle for breathing
5. Pain in the lateral neck is usually levator scapula; medially it could be splenius capitis and cervicis

II. MUSCLES THAT MOVE THE SCAPULA

A. Upward rotators (raise humerus; antagonists to downward rotators)
1. Upper trapezius
2. Lower trapezius
3. Serratus anterior

B. Downward rotators (drop humerus; antagonists to upward rotators)
1. Levator scapula
2. Rhomboids
3. Pectoralis minor

C. Elevators (raise shoulders; antagonists to depressors)
1. Upper trapezius
2. Levator scapula

D. Depressors (drop shoulders; antagonists to elevators)
1. Pectoralis minor
2. Lower trapezius

E. Protractors (roll shoulders forward; antagonists to retractors)
1. Serratus anterior
2. Pectoralis minor

F. Retractors (roll shoulders back; antagonists to protractors)
1. Middle trapezius
2. Rhomboids

G. Helpful hints
1. Serratus anterior—named for its origin on the upper-eight ribs ("ser-8-us"); strengthen by doing push-ups; weakness in this muscle causes the scapula to stick out like a chicken wing
2. Trapezius—usually involved in neck pain; the most superficial muscle of the back
3. Levator scapula—usually involved in neck and shoulder pain
4. Rhomboids—usually involved in shoulder and mid-back pain
5. Pectoralis minor—major distorter of upper body (rounded shoulders); known as an entrapper because it can compress on the axillary artery; may also be involved in entrapping the brachial plexus
6. Subclavius—helps stabilize the clavicle
7. Protraction is also known as abduction
8. Retraction is also known as adduction

III. MUSCLES THAT MOVE THE HUMERUS

A. Flexors (raise the arm overhead; antagonists to extensors)
1. Anterior deltoid
2. Pectoralis major
3. Coracobrachialis
4. Biceps (short head)

B. **Extensors (straighten the arm; antagonists to flexors)**
   1. Latissimus dorsi
   2. Teres major
   3. Posterior deltoid
   4. Infraspinatus
   5. Teres minor
   6. Triceps
   7. Pectoralis major

C. **Adductors (bring the arm toward the body; antagonists to abductors)**
   1. Pectoralis major
   2. Coracobrachialis
   3. Latissimus dorsi
   4. Teres major

D. **Abductors (move arm away from the body; antagonists to adductors)**
   1. Supraspinatus
   2. Middle deltoid

E. **Internal (medial) rotators (roll the head of the humerus forward; antagonists to external rotators)**
   1. Anterior deltoid
   2. Pectoralis major
   3. Subscapularis
   4. Teres major
   5. Latissimus dorsi

F. **External (lateral) rotators (roll the head of the humerus back; antagonists to internal rotators)**
   1. Infraspinatus
   2. Teres minor
   3. Posterior deltoid

G. **Helpful hints**
   1. Latissimus dorsi—widest muscle of the back; primary muscle used in swimming, swinging an ax, and using crutches; involved in back pain
   2. Teres major—deep to latissimus
   3. Pectoralis major—large muscle of the chest; forms the anterior aspect of the armpit (axilla)
   4. The latissimus, teres major, and pectoralis major share a common insertion; remember: "two majors and a miss"
   5. Deltoid—rounded mass of shoulder; can abduct arm to 90 degrees
   6. Coracobrachialis—named for O & I; shares a common attachment with pectoralis minor and biceps brachii (short head)
   7. Triceps—named for its three heads; only the long head extends the humerus

IV. MUSCLES THAT MOVE THE ELBOW

A. Flexors (bring forearm toward upper arm; antagonists to extensors)

1. Brachialis
2. Biceps
3. Brachioradialis

B. Extensors (straighten elbow; antagonists to flexors)

1. Triceps
2. Anconeus

C. Helpful Hints

1. Brachialis—strongest elbow flexor and can flex the elbow in any position
2. Biceps brachii—named for its two heads; can flex the elbow when forearm is supinated but when hand is pronated, does not work well
3. Brachioradialis—named for O & I; known as the "beer drinker's" muscle; works well to flex the elbow in the neutral position; makes up the lateral part of the forearm

V. MUSCLES THAT MOVE THE WRIST

A. Flexors (move fingers toward palm; antagonists to extensors)

1. Flexor carpi radialis
2. Flexor carpi ulnaris
3. Palmaris longus

B. Extensors (move fingers away from palm; antagonists to flexors)

1. Extensor carpi radialis longus
2. Extensor carpi radialis brevis
3. Extensor carpi ulnaris

C. Adductors (move hand toward the body; antagonists to abductors)

1. Extensor carpi ulnaris
2. Flexor carpi ulnaris

D. Abductors (move hand away from the body; antagonists to adductors)

1. Flexor carpi radialis
2. Extensor carpi radialis longus

E. Helpful hints

1. Carpi means wrist
2. The muscles of the forearm can be categorized into two compartments
   a) Anterior—flexor carpi ulnaris/radialis, flexor digitorum superficialis/profundus (ulnar and median nerve), palmaris longus, flexor pollicis longus; all are supplied by the median nerve except flexor carpi ulnaris (ulnar nerve)

b) Posterior—extensor carpi radialis longus/brevis, extensor carpi ulnaris, extensor digitorum, extensor digiti minimi, extensor pollicis longus/brevis; all are supplied by the radial nerve

3. There are three flexors/three extensors, two adductors/two abductors, two supinators/two pronators
4. The carpal tunnel is a passageway for the flexor tendons and the median nerve; when the flexor tendons become inflamed (overuse, entrapment), the median nerve is compressed, causing pain, numbness, tingling etc.; the flexor retinaculum holds all of the flexor tendons in place and can contribute to further compression when the flexor tendons are inflamed; this is known as carpal tunnel syndrome; hyperextension of the wrist may result in carpal tunnel syndrome also
5. The extensor retinaculum compresses the extensor tendons and holds them in place
6. Remember the ulna is the medial forearm bone and the radius is the lateral forearm bone (anatomical position)

VI. MUSCLES THAT MOVE THE FINGERS

A. Flexors (move fingers toward palm; antagonists to extensors)
1. Flexor digitorum superficialis/profundus
2. Flexor pollicis longus (flexes thumb)

B. Extensors (straighten the hand; antagonists to flexors)
1. Extensor digitorum
2. Extensor digiti minimi (little finger)
3. Extensor pollicis longus/brevis

C. Helpful hints
1. The thenar eminence is the meaty part of the thumb
2. The hypothenar eminence is the meaty part of the palm opposite the thenar eminence
3. Digit means finger
4. Pollicis means thumb
5. Opponens pollicis—responsible for opposition of the thumb (bringing the thumb over to the little finger)
6. Minimi means little

VII. MUSCLES THAT MOVE THE FOREARM

A. Supinators (turn palms up; antagonists to pronators)
1. Biceps
2. Supinator

B. Pronators (turn palms down; antagonists to supinators)
1. Pronator teres
2. Pronator quadratus

VIII. ROTATOR CUFF

A. Remember the acronym *SITS*
1. Supraspinatus
2. Infraspinatus
3. Teres minor
4. Subscapularis

B. Helpful hints
1. The actions of these muscles together allow for circumduction of the head of the humerus
2. Supraspinatus, infraspinatus and teres minor all insert on the greater tubercle of the humerus (superior, middle, inferior facets), and subscapularis inserts on the lesser tubercle

IX. MUSCLES THAT MOVE THE TRUNK

A. Flexors (make the body bend forward; antagonists to extensors)
1. Rectus abdominis
2. External oblique (bilaterally)
3. Internal oblique (bilaterally)

B. Extensors (make the trunk stay upright; antagonists to flexors)
1. Erector spinae
2. Transversospinalis

C. Rotation of trunk to opposite side
1. External oblique
2. Transversospinalis

D. Rotation of trunk to same side
1. Internal oblique

E. Lateral flexion (side bending)
1. External oblique (unilaterally)
2. Internal oblique (unilaterally)
3. Quadratus lumborum (also raises the hip, therefore nicknamed "hip hiker")

F. Helpful Hints
1. The rectus abdominis is the most superficial of the abdominal muscles
2. The linea alba (white line) runs down the center of the rectus abdominus
3. Erector spinae group from medial to lateral: spinalis, longissimus, iliocostalis
4. Transversospinalis (semispinalis, multifidus, and rotatores)
5. Weak abdominals directly contributes to chronic low back pain
6. If your trunk is turned to the left, the right external oblique and left internal oblique are contracted

7. If your trunk is turned to the right, the left external oblique and right internal oblique are contracted
8. The abdominals from deep to superficial: transverse abdominis, internal oblique, external oblique, rectus abdominis
9. The transverse abdominis runs horizontal, helps to compress the abdominal contents, and aids in forced expiration

X. MUSCLES THAT MOVE THE RIBS

A. Elevators (raise the ribs during inspiration; antagonists to depressors)
1. External intercostals
2. Scalenes (forced inspiration)
3. SCM (accessory respiratory muscle)
4. Pectoralis minor (accessory respiratory muscle)
5. Quadratus lumborum

B. Depressors (lower the ribs during expiration; antagonists to elevators)
1. Internal intercostals
2. Abdominals
3. Quadratus lumborum

C. Helpful hints
1. The QL assists in respiration because of its attachment on the 12th rib
2. The diaphragm is the most significant muscle used in breathing

XI. MUSCLES THAT MOVE THE FEMUR

A. Hip flexors (bring the femur upward; antagonists to extensors)
1. Iliopsoas (psoas)
2. Pectineus
3. Tensor fasciae latae
4. Adductors (brevis, longus, magnus)
5. Rectus femoris
6. Sartorius

B. Hip extensors (bring the femur back to neutral; antagonists to flexors)
1. Gluteus maximus
2. Hamstrings

C. Abductors (lift leg away from the midline; antagonists to adductors)
1. Gluteus medius
2. Gluteus minimus
3. Tensor fasciae latae
4. Sartorius

D. Adductors (bring leg toward the midline; antagonists to abductors)
1. Adductors (brevis, longus, magnus)

2. Gracilis
3. Pectineus

E. **External (lateral) rotators (antagonists to internal rotators)**
1. Deep six
2. Gluteus maximus
3. Iliopsoas
4. Sartorius

F. **Internal (medial) rotators (antagonists to external rotators)**
1. Gluteus medius
2. Gluteus minimus
3. Tensor fasciae latae
4. Pectineus
5. Adductors (brevis, longus, magnus)

G. **Helpful hints**
1. Iliopsoas is commonly referred to as the psoas; psoas is the strongest hip flexor
2. Hypercontraction of the psoas will result in a person being stooped over
3. Rectus femoris is the only quadricep that crosses two joints
4. Sartorius is the longest muscle in the body
5. Gluteus maximus is known as the "power muscle"—used in climbing stairs, running, raising from a seated position
6. Hamstrings—medial to lateral: semimembranosus, semitendinosus, and biceps femoris; biceps femoris has two heads, so there are four heads in the hamstring group; all hamstrings cross two joints (knee and hip); semitendinosus inserts on the anterior aspect of the tibia
7. External (lateral) rotators—the toes point away from the midline
8. Internal (medial) rotators—toes are pointed toward the midline
9. Deep six—piriformis (*strongest lateral hip rotator*), gemellus superior/inferior, obturator externus/internus, quadratus femoris
10. Piriformis is known as an entrapper because it can entrap the sciatic nerve
11. The sciatic nerve runs through the sciatic notch and is palpated deep in the gluteal region

XII. MUSCLES THAT MOVE THE KNEE

A. **Flexors (bend the knee; antagonists to extensors)**
1. Hamstrings
2. Sartorius
3. Gracilis
4. Gastrocnemius
5. Plantaris
6. Popliteus

B. **Extensors (straighten the knee; antagonists to flexors)**
1. Quadriceps
2. Tensor fasciae latae

C. Helpful hints
1. Gastrocnemius has two heads
2. Popliteus allows for the knee to bend by "unlocking" it
3. Quadriceps—vastus lateralis/intermedius/medialis, rectus femoris

XIII. MUSCLES THAT MOVE THE ANKLE

A. Dorsiflexors (bring toes toward the leg; antagonists to plantar-flexors)
1. Tibialis anterior
2. Extensor digitorum longus
3. Extensor hallucis longus
4. Peroneus tertius

B. Plantar-flexors (toes away from the leg; antagonists to dorsi-flexors)
1. Soleus
2. Gastrocnemius
3. Plantaris
4. Peroneus longus and brevis
5. Tibialis posterior
6. Flexor hallucis longus
7. Flexor digitorum longus

C. Invertors (antagonists to evertors)
1. Tibialis anterior
2. Tibialis posterior

D. Evertors (antagonists to invertors)
1. Peroneus longus
2. Peroneus brevis
3. Peroneus tertius

E. Helpful hints
1. The leg is divided into the anterior, posterior and lateral compartments
    a) Anterior—tibialis anterior, extensor hallucis longus, extensor digitorum longus, and peroneus tertius; all dorsiflex the foot and are supplied by the peroneal nerve
    b) Posterior—superficial: gastrocnemius, soleus, plantaris; deep: tibialis posterior, flexor digitorum longus, flexor hallucis longus; all are supplied by the tibial nerve
    c) Lateral—peroneus longus, peroneus brevis
2. The anterior and posterior compartments are opposite of each other (tibialis anterior/posterior, extensor digitorum/flexor digitorum, extensor hallucis/flexor hallucis)
3. Hallucis means big toe
4. Digit means finger or toe (excluding thumb and big toe)
5. Paralysis of the tibialis anterior will cause "drop foot"
6. Dorsiflexion—also known as extension
7. Plantar-flexion—also known as flexion

8. Gastrocnemius—the muscle involved in pain from wearing high heels
9. Gastrocnemius, soleus, and plantaris tendons make up the Achilles (calcaneal) tendon
10. Injury to the tibialis anterior and/or posterior causes shin splints; shin splints involve the periosteum around the tibia
11. Invertors roll the ankle so the soles of the feet are facing each other
12. Evertors roll the ankle so the soles of the feet are facing away from the body
13. Peroneal means fibula; all peroneal muscles are on the lateral compartment of the leg

XIV. MUSCLES THAT MOVE THE TOES

A. **Flexors (point the toes toward the floor; antagonists to extensors)**
   1. Flexor digitorum longus
   2. Flexor hallucis

B. **Extensors (bring the toes toward the body; antagonists to flexors)**
   1. Extensor digitorum longus
   2. Extensor hallucis longus

XV. OTHER MUSCLES

A. **Masseter**—responsible for raising and protracting the mandible

B. **Temporalis**—elevates and retracts the mandible

C. **Pes anseurinus**—common tendon insertion of the semitendinosus, gracilis, and sartorius

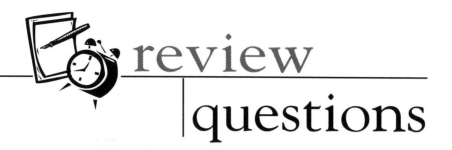
review questions

DIRECTIONS Each of the questions or incomplete statements below is followed by suggested answers or completions. Select the one answer that is best in each case.

1. The hamstring muscles from medial to lateral are:
   A. Biceps femoris, semitendinosus, semi-membranosus.
   B. Semitendinosus, semimembranosus, biceps femoris.
   C. Semimembranosus, semitendinosus, rectus femoris.
   D. Semimembranosus, semitendinosus, biceps femoris.

2. A client presents with chronic low back pain. Which muscle would be weak?
   A. Rectus abdominis
   B. Quadratus lumborum
   C. Latissimus dorsi
   D. Rhomboid

3. If the psoas muscle is hypercontracted (chronic) which postural deviation will occur?
   A. Stoop
   B. Sway-back
   C. Short-arm syndrome
   D. Shin splints

4. Where do you palpate the sciatic notch?
   A. Deep in the adductor region
   B. Deep in the gluteal region
   C. Deep in the femoral region
   D. Deep in the inguinal region

5. Which is the best position to place your client in to palpate the vastus medialis?
   A. Seated
   B. Side-lying
   C. Supine
   D. Prone

6. How would you help a client to strengthen the rhomboids?
   A. Have the client sit on floor and flex the elbow.
   B. Have the client lie prone and resist abduction of the arm.
   C. Have the client lie supine and resist supination of the forearm.
   D. Have the client lie prone with arms off table and retract the shoulder blades.

7. Which muscle can entrap the brachial plexus?
   A. Scalenes
   B. Temporalis
   C. Triceps
   D. Deltoids

8. Which movement brings the arm closer to the midline?
   A. Abduction
   B. Adduction
   C. Circumduction
   D. Supination

9. A client reports their toenails are putting holes in their shoes. Which muscle is likely to be involved?
    A. Extensor carpi radialis
    B. Extensor digitorum longus
    C. Extensor carpi ulnaris
    D. Extensor digitorum tertius

10. Which anterior muscle would you work for a client that suffers from lordosis?
    A. Pectoralis major
    B. Vastus medialis
    C. Iliopsoas
    D. Diaphragm

11. Which muscle is involved in normal respiration?
    A. Intercostals
    B. External oblique
    C. SCM
    D. Scalenes

12. If a MT hyperextends her wrist, what may result?
    A. TMJ
    B. Carpal tunnel syndrome
    C. Peroneal muscle sprain
    D. Rupture of the inguinal ligament

13. The biceps femoris performs these two actions:
    A. Extension and medial rotation.
    B. Flexion and medial rotation.
    C. Extension and abduction.
    D. Flexion and extension.

14. A client reports having whiplash and the brachial plexus is impinged. Which muscle is likely to be involved?
    A. Deltoids
    B. Pectoralis minor
    C. Rhomboids
    D. Triceps

15. In Western anatomical position, the ulna is the _____ forearm bone.
    A. Lateral
    B. Medial
    C. Contralateral
    D. Ipsilateral

16. Which muscle flexes the knee and extends the hip?
    A. Rectus femoris
    B. Semitendinosus
    C. Gluteus maximus
    D. Gastrocnemius

17. Which muscle is shortened when a person is wearing high heel shoes?
    A. Tibialis anterior
    B. Peroneus tertius
    C. Popliteus
    D. Gastrocnemius

18. A client comes in for a massage and the scapula is still abducted after the massage. Which muscle do you recommend that the client stretch?
    A. Pectoralis minor
    B. Rhomboids
    C. Subscapularis
    D. Latissimus dorsi

19. What do you call the bony prominence at the proximal end of the ulna?
    A. Medial epicondyle
    B. Lateral epicondyle
    C. Olecranon process
    D. Styloid process

20. When massaging the lateral head of the fibula, of which structure should you be careful?
    A. Popliteal endangerment site
    B. Peroneal nerve
    C. Tibial nerve
    D. Femoral nerve

21. Compression on the sciatic nerve by which muscle causes pain and tingling that radiates down the posterior leg?
    A. Scalene.
    B. Popliteus.
    C. Plantaris.
    D. Piriformis.

22. With your client in the supine position, how do you expose the serratus anterior?
    A. Lateral rotation and adduction of the arm
    B. Medial rotation and adduction of the arm
    C. Horizontal abduction of the arm
    D. Horizontal adduction of the arm

23. The primary muscle involved in running downhill is the:
    A. Quadriceps.
    B. Hamstrings.
    C. Peroneus tertius.
    D. Opponens longus.

24. Hypercontraction of the pectoralis minor causes rounded shoulders. Which muscle would be weak and overstretched?
    A. Pectoralis minor
    B. Rhomboids
    C. Subclavius
    D. Levator scapula

25. The muscles that make up the rotator cuff are:
    A. Supraspinatus, infraspinatus, teres major, subscapularis.
    B. Supraspinatus, infraspinatus, teres minor, serratus anterior.
    C. Supraspinatus, infraspinatus, teres major, serratus anterior.
    D. Supraspinatus, infraspinatus, teres minor, subscapularis.

26. A synergist to the teres major is:
    A. Supraspinatus.
    B. Rhomboids.
    C. Latissimus dorsi.
    D. Pectoralis minor.

27. All of these muscles share a common attachment:
    A. Biceps brachii, brachioradialis, coracobrachialis.
    B. Coracobrachialis, brachioradialis, pectoralis minor.
    C. Pectoralis minor, coracobrachialis, brachioradialis.
    D. Biceps brachii, coracobrachialis, pectoralis minor.

28. The linea aspera is on the posterior:
    A. Tibia.
    B. Femur.
    C. Ischium.
    D. Humerus.

29. The acromion process is on the superior aspect of the:
    A. Scapula.
    B. Sternum.
    C. Clavicle.
    D. Humerus.

30. Which muscle laterally rotates the knee?
    A. Semitendinosus.
    B. Rectus femoris.
    C. Vastus medialis.
    D. Biceps femoris.

31. All of the following dorsiflex the ankle except:
    A. Tibialis anterior.
    B. Extensor hallucis longus.
    C. Peroneus longus.
    D. Peroneus tertius.

32. Which muscle crosses both the knee and the ankle and is a strong plantarflexor?
    A. Tibialis posterior.
    B. Peroneus brevis.
    C. Gastrocnemius.
    D. Soleus.

33. Which muscle is involved in shin splints?
    A. Soleus.
    B. Tibialis posterior.

C. Popliteus.

D. Plantaris.

34. The white line of the abdominal fascia is known as the:

A. Linea alba.

B. Inguinal ligament.

C. Abdominal aponeurosis.

D. Rectus abdominis.

35. The action of the deltoid muscles working as a group is:

A. Extension.

B. Adduction.

C. Abduction.

D. Flexion.

36. In muscle contraction, the greatest amount of movement takes place at the:

A. Origin.

B. Insertion.

C. Belly.

D. Extensor.

37. Which muscle stabilizes the scapula by preventing extreme elevation and protraction of the clavicle?

A. Subscapularis

B. Subclavius

C. Supraspinatus

D. Serratus anterior

38. The widest muscle of the back is:

A. Latissimus dorsi.

B. Trapezius.

C. Teres major.

D. Erector spinae.

39. Which muscle supinates the forearm?

A. Pronator quadratus

B. Triceps brachii

C. Biceps brachii

D. Brachioradialis

40. Which abdominal muscle rotates the trunk to the same side?

A. External oblique.

B. Internal oblique.

C. Rectus abdominis.

D. Transverse abdominis.

41. The strongest elbow flexor is:

A. Brachioradialis.

B. Biceps brachii.

C. Coracobrachialis.

D. Brachialis.

42. The action of the triceps as a group is:

A. Extension of the humerus.

B. Extension of the elbow.

C. Flexion of the elbow.

D. Flexion of the humerus.

43. Flexors of the humerus are:

A. Coracobrachialis, biceps, triceps.

B. Infraspinatus, teres minor, pectoralis minor.

C. Pectoralis major, biceps, triceps.

D. Biceps, coracobrachialis, pectoralis major.

44. Which is not an attachment of the SCM?

A. Styloid process

B. Mastoid process

C. Medial clavicle

D. Manubrium of the sternum

45. The muscle that does not attach to the humerus is:

A. Pectoralis major.   C. Subscapularis.

B. Biceps brachii.   D. Brachialis.

46. Which of the following is not a wrist extensor?

A. Extensor carpi radialis longus

B. Extensor carpi radialis brevis

C. Extensor carpi ulnaris

D. Extensor digitorum

47. The tendons that make up the Pes anseurinus are:

A. Semitendinosus, semimembranosus, gracilis.

B. Semimembranosus, gracilis, sartorius.

C. Sartorius, gracilis, semimembranosus.

D. Gracilis, semitendinosus, sartorius.

48. The longest muscle in the body is:
    A. Great saphenous.
    B. Gracilis.
    C. Sartorius.
    D. Pectineus.

49. Which of the following muscles does not attach to the bicipital groove?
    A. Pectoralis minor
    B. Latissimus dorsi
    C. Teres major
    D. Pectoralis major

50. When the humerus is rotated laterally, which muscle is stretched?
    A. Infraspinatus
    B. Teres minor
    C. Teres major
    D. Pectoralis minor

51. Which muscle rotates the head to the same side?
    A. SCM
    B. Levator scapula
    C. Upper trapezius
    D. Splenius capitis

52. Which muscle has no attachments on the scapula?
    A. Pectoralis major
    B. Subscapularis
    C. Rhomboids
    D. Pectoralis minor

53. Name the erector spinae muscles lateral to medial.
    A. Longissimus, iliocostalis, spinalis.
    B. Iliocostalis, longissimus, spinalis.
    C. Spinalis, longissimus, iliocostalis.
    D. Iliocostalis, spinalis, longissimus.

54. The functions of the erector spinae muscles are:
    A. Unilateral flexion of the spine, extension of the hip bilaterally.
    B. Bilateral flexion of the spine, flexion of the hip unilaterally.

C. Bilateral extension of the spine, lateral flexion of the spine.
D. Unilateral extension of the spine, bilateral flexion of the spine.

55. Which two muscles are involved in a lateral ankle sprain?
    A. Peroneus longus and brevis
    B. Tibialis anterior and posterior
    C. Flexor and extensor digitorum longus
    D. Gastrocnemius and soleus

56. Which muscles invert the foot?
    A. Peroneus longus and brevis
    B. Tibialis anterior and posterior
    C. Flexor and extensor digitorum longus
    D. Gastrocnemius and soleus

57. A client reports having broken the distal aspect of their shoulder. Which joint would have been involved?
    A. Acromioclavicular
    B. Sternoclavicular
    C. Radioulnar
    D. Acetabulofemoral

58. The correct medical nomenclature for the bony prominence commonly called the ankle is:
    A. Epicondyle.
    B. Malleoli.
    C. Phalanges.
    D. Condyle.

59. A Colle's fracture would involve which bone?
    A. Ulna
    B. Radius
    C. Fibula
    D. Tibia

60. A Pott's fracture would involve which bone?
    A. Ulna
    B. Radius
    C. Fibula
    D. Tibia

61. Which muscle would be most fatigued after the completion of a 50-kilometer bike race?
    A. Hamstrings
    B. Popliteus
    C. Trapezius
    D. Quadriceps

62. The origin of the gluteus maximus is:
    A. Superior gluteal line.
    B. Middle gluteal line.
    C. Inferior gluteal line.
    D. Linea aspera.

63. How many heads in the hamstring group?
    A. 2
    B. 3
    C. 4
    D. 5

64. Which muscle crosses two joints?
    A. Popliteus
    B. Brachialis
    C. Soleus
    D. Rectus femoris

65. The insertion of the triceps is the:
    A. Lateral epicondyle of the humerus.
    B. Medial epicondyle of the humerus.
    C. Olecranon process of the radius.
    D. Olecranon process of the ulna.

66. Which muscle is not a hip flexor?
    A. Rectus femoris
    B. Iliopsoas
    C. Vastus lateralis
    D. Tensor fascia latae

67. All of these muscle extend the humerus except:
    A. Latissimus dorsi.
    B. Biceps brachii.
    C. Teres major.
    D. Teres minor.

68. This muscle flexes the elbow in the neutral position:
    A. Coracobrachialis.
    B. Anconeus.
    C. Brachioradialis.
    D. Triceps brachii.

69. These muscles are known as "entrappers," because when hypercontracted, they may entrap a nerve or nerve plexus:
    A. Biceps brachii, pectoralis minor, piriformis.
    B. Pectoralis major, piriformis, SCM.
    C. Scalenes, pectoralis minor, biceps brachii.
    D. Pectoralis minor, scalenes, piriformis.

70. Which muscle is part of the IT band?
    A. Iliopsoas
    B. Tensor fascia latae
    C. Semimembranosus
    D. Plantaris

71. The strongest lateral hip rotator is:
    A. Iliopsoas.
    B. Adductor magnus.
    C. Piriformis.
    D. Sartorius.

72. Which muscles are located in the femoral region?
    A. Hamstrings
    B. Quadriceps
    C. Adductors
    D. Scalenes

73. Which muscle performs only one action?
    A. Gastrocnemius
    B. Biceps brachii
    C. Biceps femoris
    D. Soleus

74. These tendons make up the Achilles tendon:
    A. Gastrocnemius and soleus.
    B. Plantaris and semitendinosus.
    C. Semitendinosus and soleus.
    D. Biceps femoris and gastrocnemius.

75. The most superficial muscle of the back is:
    A. Latissimus dorsi.
    B. Trapezius.
    C. Teres major.
    D. Teres minor.

76. Paralysis of this muscle causes drop foot:
    A. Tibialis anterior.
    B. Tibialis posterior.
    C. Popliteus.
    D. Plantaris.

77. All of the following abduct the hip except:
    A. Gluteus medius.
    B. Sartorius.
    C. Gracilis.
    D. Tensor fascia latae.

78. This muscle is both an antagonist and synergist to the rectus femoris:
    A. Tibialis posterior.
    B. Piriformis.
    C. Biceps femoris.
    D. Sartorius.

79. Which muscle would you be affecting when massaging lateral to the vastus lateralis?
    A. Pectineus
    B. Tensor fasciae latae
    C. Vastus medialis
    D. Gracilis

80. The origin of the levator scapula is:
    A. Spinous processes of C1–C4.
    B. Spine of scapula.
    C. Transverse processes of C1–C4.
    D. Coracoid process of scapula.

81. This muscle's action is elevation and downward rotation of the scapula:
    A. Levator scapula.
    B. Trapezius.
    C. Rhomboids.
    D. Teres major.

82. This muscle acts on the big toe:
    A. Adductor pollicis longus.
    B. Extensor hallucis longus.
    C. Flexor digitorum longus.
    D. Extensor digitorum longus.

83. This muscle closes the jaw:
    A. Scalene.
    B. Masseter.
    C. Frontalis.
    D. SCM.

84. Which muscle stabilizes the humerus in the glenoid cavity and abducts the humerus?
    A. Teres major
    B. Trapezius
    C. Subscapularis
    D. Supraspinatus

85. This is the primary muscle used in swimming and may become irritated from using crutches:
    A. Trapezius.
    B. Supraspinatus.
    C. Latissimus dorsi.
    D. Pectoralis minor.

86. The muscle responsible for flexion, extension and abduction of the shoulder is:
    A. Teres minor.
    B. Teres major.
    C. Biceps brachii.
    D. Deltoid.

87. The muscle that opposes the serratus anterior is:
    A. Teres major.
    B. Infraspinatus.
    C. Rhomboids major.
    D. Levator scapula.

88. Which muscle adducts the wrist?
    A. Palmaris longus
    B. Flexor carpi radialis
    C. Flexor carpi ulnaris
    D. Flexor digitorum superficialis

89. The fleshy mass at the base of the thumb is:
    A. Hypothenar eminence.
    B. Thenar eminence.
    C. Antebrachium.
    D. Extensor retinaculum.

90. If your trunk is rotated to the right, which two muscles are engaged?
    A. Right internal and left external oblique
    B. Left internal and right external oblique
    C. Right internal and right external oblique
    D. Left internal and left external oblique

91. Loss of function of the wrist and medial fingers is caused by injury of the:
    A. Ulnar nerve.
    B. Radial nerve.
    C. Peroneal nerve.
    D. Femoral nerve.

92. Spasmodic torticollis involves which muscle?
    A. Subscapularis
    B. Splenius capitis
    C. SCM
    D. External oblique

93. We do not massage the SCM bilaterally because of the:
    A. Femoral artery.
    B. Common carotid artery.
    C. Peroneal artery.
    D. Tibial artery.

94. Peroneal nerve damage diminishes the ability to:
    A. Evert the foot.
    B. Invert the foot.
    C. Pronate the arm.
    D. Supinate the arm.

95. This muscle may be strengthened by doing push-ups:
    A. Pectoralis minor.
    B. Subclavius.

C. Peroneus longus.
D. Serratus anterior.

96. This muscle abducts the wrist:
    A. Extensor carpi radialis longus.
    B. Extensor carpi ulnaris.
    C. Extensor digitorum.
    D. Palmaris longus.

97. The muscle(s) located in the posterior femoral region is/are:
    A. Quadriceps.
    B. Hamstrings.
    C. Triceps surae.
    D. Triceps brachii.

98. The muscle of the rotator cuff responsible for medial rotation is:
    A. Supraspinatus.
    B. Infraspinatus.
    C. Teres minor.
    D. Subscapularis.

99. This muscle brings the arm forward:
    A. Coracobrachialis.
    B. Latissimus dorsi.
    C. Infraspinatus.
    D. Teres minor.

100. This muscle initiates walking:
    A. Gluteus medius.
    B. Iliopsoas.
    C. Semimembranosus.
    D. Tibialis posterior.

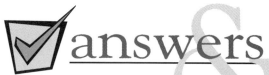

answers & rationales

The answer key will give you two pieces of information. The first is the correct answer, the second is the rationale.

1.
D. Remember semimembranosus—m for medial

2.
A. Key word—weak (indicates the antagonist)

3.
A. When contracted, the iliopsoas raises the femur; if the client is upright, this would cause forward stoop

4.
B. Remember where the sciatic nerve runs

5.
C. The vastus medialis is part of the quadriceps group

6.
D. The rhomboids retract the scapula

7.
A. The other "entrappers" are the piriformis and pectoralis minor

8.
B. Abduction—away from the midline

9.
B. Extensor carpi radialis and ulnaris are on the arm; D is not a muscle

10.
C. The iliopsoas is the only opposing muscle listed as a choice

11.
A. Key words—normal respiration

12.
B. Hyperextension would cause increased pressure on the flexor retinaculum

13.
D. Extension of hip and flexion of the knee

14.
B. Pectoralis minor and the scalenes can entrap the brachial plexus

15.
B. Anatomical position—upright with palms facing forward

16.
B. All three hamstrings perform these actions

17.
D. The foot will be plantar-flexed when wearing high heels

18.
A. The pectoralis minor is an antagonist to the rhomboids

19.
C. Attachment site for the triceps

20.
B. Key word—lateral; peroneal means fibula

21.
D. Known as an entrapper because it can entrap the sciatic nerve

22.
C. Horizontal adduction would bring the arm across the body

23.
A. Hamstrings would provide force in running uphill by extending the hip

24.
B. Rhomboids are an antagonist to the pectoralis minor

25.
D. Key—teres minor

26.
C. They both adduct and extend the humerus

27.
D. They all attach to the coracoid process of the scapula

28.
B. The origin for the biceps femoris

29.
A. The bony projection on the top of the shoulder

30.
D. Located on the lateral aspect of the thigh

31.
C. Inserts on the medial plantar surface of the foot

32.
C. Key—crosses both joints

33.
B. Both tibialis anterior and posterior are involved in shinsplints

34.
A. Literally means "white line"

35.
C. All three of the muscles work together to abduct the humerus

36.
B. The origin is the most stable part of the muscle

37.
B. Basically its only function

38.
A. The trapezius is the most superficial

39.
C. The supinator and the biceps supinate the forearm

40.
B. External obliques rotate the trunk to the opposite side

41.
D. Works to flex the elbow in any position

42.
B. Only the long head of the triceps extends the humerus

43.
D. Triceps and teres minor extend the humerus

44.
A. Named for its origin and insertion: sterno—sternum, cleido—clavicle, mastoid—mastoid process

45.
B. Origin—scapula; insertion—radius

46.
D. Key words—extensor of the wrist

47.
D. All insert on the anterior tibia

48.
C. Great saphenous is the longest vein

49.
A. Origin—coracoid process; insertion—ribs

50.
C. Teres major medially rotates the humerus

51.
D. SCM rotates the head to the opposite side

52.
A. Origin—clavicle, sternum; insertion—bicipital groove

53.
B. Named for location: iliocostalis—ribs, longissimus—middle, spinalis—spine

54.
C. Bilateral—both sides; unilateral—one side

55.
A. Peroneal means fibula—the lateral leg bone

56.
B. Both insert on the medial aspect of the foot

57.
A. Named for its location: acromio (acromion), clavicular (clavicle)

58.
B. Plural for malleolus

59.
B. Pott's fracture involves the fibula

60.
C. Colles' fracture involves the radius

61.
D. Power to push the pedals comes from the quadriceps

62.
A. Gluteus medius—middle; gluteus minimus—inferior

63.
C. Two heads for the biceps femoris

64.
D. Hip and knee

65.
D. All three heads insert here

66.
C. The vastus lateralis does not cross the hip joint

67.
B. All of the other choices are on the posterior of the body

68.
C. Coracobrachialis flexes the humerus

69.
D. Pectoralis minor; axillary artery/brachial plexus; scalenes—brachial plexus; piriformis—sciatic nerve

70.
B. The TFL and the IT tract are often referred to as the IT band

71.
C. It is listed first in the text, it is the strongest

72.
C. Femoral region is the pubic area

73.
D. Only performs plantar-flexion of the ankle

74.
A. The only two choices listed in the posterior leg

75.
B. Latissimus is the widest

76.
A. Foot drop is when the foot is in plantar-flexion. Tibialis anterior is the only muscle listed that is a dorsiflexor

77.
C. Gracilis is an adductor of the femur

78.
D. Flexes the hip and flexes the knee

79.
B. On the lateral aspect of the thigh

80.
C. Insertion is the root of the spine of the scapula

81.
A. The trapezius rotates the scapula upward

82.
B. Hallucis—big toe; pollicis—thumb

83.
B. Closes and protracts the mandible

84.
D. The only two actions this muscle performs

85.
C. The strongest extensor of the humerus

86.
D. None of the other choices abducts the humerus

87.
C. Serratus protracts the scapula; the rhomboids retract

88.
C. The only choice with "ulna" in it

89.
B. Key words—base of the thumb

90.
A. External obliques turn the trunk to the opposite side; internal—same side

91.
A. Key words—medial fingers; ulna is the medial arm bone

92.
C. Think of a tortoise neck

93.
B. All of the other choices are in the lower body

94.
A. Peroneal muscles evert the foot

95.
D. Doing push-ups will affect both the origin and insertion

96.
A. The only choice with "radius" in it

97.
B. Key words: posterior femoral

98.
D. All the other choices laterally rotate the humerus

99.
A. All the other choices extend the humerus

100.
B. The only muscle listed that flexes the femur

4

Massage and the Business of Massage

contents

I. MASSAGE

A. **Massage is defined as the manual manipulation of the soft tissues of the body**
   1. The most widely recognized benefits of massage are relaxation, improved blood and lymphatic circulation, and pain management

B. **Massage disappeared during the Middle Ages and reappeared during the Renaissance**

C. **Effects and benefits of massage**
   1. *Psychological*—relaxation and improved well-being
   2. *Mechanical*—improves blood/lymph flow, breaks up adhesions/scar tissue, lengthens/stretches muscles and fascia, and increases range of motion (ROM)
   3. *Physiological*—improves functioning at the cellular level, brings blood to the area (hyperemia), decreases pain by resetting nociceptors (pain receptors), assists in the removal of metabolic wastes and encourages release of natural endorphins (painkillers)

D. **Strokes**
   1. *Effleurage* (gliding strokes)—may be superficial or deep
      a) Gentle stroking directed toward the heart (centripetal)
      b) Assists in tissue assessment, determining pain tolerance level of the client, distributes lubricant, allows the client to become accustomed to the therapist's touch
      c) Beginning and end strokes of the massage
      d) Most widely used stroke in massage
      e) Slow, rhythmic stroking will affect the parasympathetic nervous system by decreasing heart rate and for a short time, blood pressure
      f) Deep stroking will assist in venous/lymph return, stretch muscles and fascia (remember: muscular contraction, breathing, elevation above the heart of the extremity, and manual manipulations assist venous return)
      g) Effleurage will help to reduce edema in the extremities; always massage above the edemic area first (hip, thigh, leg then the feet if the edema is in the feet)
      h) Used as a "connecting" stroke
      i) Can use hands, fingers, and/or arms to apply effleurage
   2. *Petrissage* (kneading)—lifts and separates tissue
      a) Milks the tissue of metabolic waste
      b) Includes compression, rolling, and skin-rolling
      c) Improves circulation by assisting venous and lymph return
      d) Separates muscle fibers
      e) Promotes relaxation
      f) Decreases adhesions in the tissue
      g) Promotes hyperemia to the area being worked on
   3. *Friction* (cross-fiber/transverse or circular)
      a) Promotes hyperemia/heat in the tissue

b) Used in the sub-acute or chronic stage of an injury

c) Promotes healing

d) Breaks down adhesions/scar tissue

e) Moves superficial layer of tissue against deeper layers and usually over/against a structural surface (bone)

f) Can be used in muscle belly or over tendons and ligaments

g) Compression, rolling (rapid back and forth movement), chucking (moving the flesh up and down over the bone), wringing (hands work in opposite directions), and shaking (to loosen and release tension)

h) Creates the most heat in the tissue because it is the deepest stroke

i) Rolling may be used to warm up a body part quickly

4. *Tapotement*

a) Hacking, cupping, slapping, tapping, clapping, rapping, and pincement

b) Initially stimulating then relaxing after prolonged application

c) Used to loosen phlegm and increase mucal secretions over the thoracic area, improve circulation in an amputee's stump, and stimulation at the end of the massage to assist in waking up your client

d) Three stages—stimulating, relaxing, sedating

5. *Vibration*

a) Light (used to leave an area of the body after finishing effleurage strokes)

b) Mechanical (vibrators) thumping or circular

c) Used over nerve trunks or centers

d) Includes shaking and jostling

E. Contraindications

1. Definition—treatment is inadvisable or course of treatment is not recommended

2. All pathologies should be considered when deciding to massage a client or not

3. If you are unsure if a treatment is contraindicated or not, reschedule the appointment and do more research or contact your clients physician for approval

4. Never proceed with the massage if you are uncertain of the pathologies

5. Always refer your client to appropriate professionals

6. Never work outside your scope of practice

7. Using too much pressure while performing deep strokes will cause the muscle to cramp

F. Endangerment sites

1. An area of concern that may contain underlying structures that could be damaged through massage

a) Groove inferior to ear—styloid process

    b) Anterior triangle—carotid, jugular arteries and vagus nerve

    c) Posterior triangle—brachial plexus, subclavian artery

    d) Axilla (armpit)—axillary, median, ulnar nerves, axillary artery, lymph nodes

    e) Ulnar notch—ulnar nerve

    f) Femoral triangle—femoral artery, nerve, vein, great saphenous vein, inguinal ligament, lymph nodes

    g) Popliteal area (behind the knee)—popliteal artery, nerve; tibial, peroneal nerve

    h) Abdomen—aorta, R-liver/gallbladder, L-spleen/stomach

    i) Lumbar—kidneys

    j) Cubital—median, radial, ulnar arteries

    k) Medial brachium—ulnar, median nerves; brachial artery

II. PERFORMING THE MASSAGE

A. The massage environment

1. Temperature should be comfortable for your client, not what you want
2. Clean linens are always used and washed after each use
3. Clean table in between clients
4. Always wash hands and keep nails short and clean
5. Be aware of personal hygiene/body odor, including breath, cigarette smoke, perfume, scented lotions, etc.
6. Always consult with your client before the use of aromatherapy and music
7. Treatment area should be clear of all clutter
8. Lighting should be subdued and preferably not from overhead lights
9. When using oil as a lubricant, it should be water-soluble so it doesn't stain your sheets
10. Do not use mineral oils; they clog pores
11. Treatment room should be ventilated

B. Bolstering

1. Always bolster so that your client is comfortable
2. A bolster under the knees when your client is supine will take pressure off the low back
3. A flat bolster/pillow under the abdomen will alleviate pressure from the low back when client is prone
4. Bolsters/towels under the anterior shoulder region when client is prone will help alleviate pressure on chest for large-breasted women or those with extreme protraction of scapula
5. A bolster under the ankles when client is prone will assist in venous flow
6. A bolster/pillow between the legs will take pressure off the pelvic joints when side-lying
7. When client is side-lying, bolster/pillow under head and under arm for comfort

C. The massage

1. If the client is not a regular, always ask if this is your client's first massage
2. Be prepared with questions/answers to client's questions
3. Explain the massage procedure to your client prior to them disrobing and getting on the table
4. Do not allow your client to disrobe in front of you; leave the room and give them privacy
5. Have all of your products/supplies ready before the client arrives
6. Adjust the table for the size of the client, type of massage, and practitioner's height
7. Assist or explain for your client how to get on and off the table
8. Always maintain your client's dignity by draping appropriately; at all times, the pelvic area will be draped
9. A diaper drape is used to cover all parts of the trunk except the appendages
10. Be flexible; this is your client's massage, not yours; adhere to clients' requests as long as they are within your scope of practice
11. Continually monitor your client throughout the massage; if you notice changes in breathing, tension, etc., talk to your client and adjust your massage accordingly
12. If your client becomes emotional during the massage, ask if you should continue
13. Treat your clients with empathy, not sympathy
14. If while performing the massage, you come across a pathology you are not sure of, stop the massage, and wash your hands; if necessary, reschedule the appointment so you can further research the pathology and/or contact the client's physician
15. If you feel uncomfortable with the way a client is acting, say something immediately; *silence is acceptance*
16. If during the massage, the client is inappropriate, stop the massage and tell the client why you stopped the massage
17. At the end of the massage, tell your client that the massage is complete and give instructions on how to get off the table slowly (roll onto side); after the client dresses, you will meet the client in the common area
18. After the massage, encourage client to drink water
19. Encourage your client to contact his or her physician if during the massage you discovered a pathology the client was not aware of
20. Posture and body mechanics are extremely important—not just to deliver a good massage, but for protection against injury; keep body weight evenly distributed on feet, rocking from front foot to back foot when necessary; keep elbows close to body; power comes from the core of the body, not the arms and shoulders

D. Infection control and safety

1. Protect yourself and your client by exercising universal precautions

2. Wash hands and arms before and after each massage
3. Always ask your clients prior to the massage if they have any open wounds, sores, blemishes, rashes etc., and avoid the area during the massage
4. Immediately stop and wash hands during the massage if you come in contact with an open wound, rash, or an unknown blemish on the skin
5. If a client has particularly dirty (or odorous) feet or hands, you may choose to avoid the area completely, explaining why or perform that portion of the massage through the linens
6. Wear latex gloves when necessary
7. Do not cross-contaminate products; when working from bulk products, use a spoon, knife, etc., to take out what you need; do not use your fingers
8. Keep nails short and clean
9. Keep your treatment room/area clean and free of clutter
10. Ask your clients to shower before coming in for their appointment
11. Above all, use common sense in working to protect you and your client

E. First aid/CPR

1. Every therapist should be certified in basic first aid/CPR whether required by law or not
2. Always call for advanced life-support *first* then begin your intervention
3. If a client appears to be suffering from a heart attack (*myocardial infarction*) or stroke (*cerebrovascular accident; CVA*) call 911 and begin the basic life support ABCs—A (airway), B (breathing), C (circulation)
4. If a client is choking, encourage him/her to continue coughing; when the victim can no longer cough or passes out, you need to perform first aid for choking; if the client passes out, contact 911 and continue to try to dislodge the obstruction
5. If a client feels faint, have the person lay down, loosen clothing around his or her neck, elevate the client's legs; you can also have the client sit in a chair with his or her head hanging down between his or her knees
6. *Heat cramps*—the client experiences muscle cramps, heavy perspiration; move to a cool area, give water and do not massage
7. *Heat exhaustion*—the clients skin is cold, heavy perspiration; move the client to a cool area, elevate legs, seek medical attention
8. *Heat stroke*—life threatening; the client is not sweating; skin is dry; move the client to a cool area, elevate head/shoulders, and call medical staff immediately
9. *Strain*—includes the muscle and is painful; weakness may occur; apply RICE (universal treatment for sprains/strains)—R-rest, I-ice, C-compression, E-elevation
10. *Sprains*—involves the musculotendinous unit; joint becomes hypermobile and deformed; seek professional help

III. HYDROTHERAPY

A. The use of water in a solid state (ice), liquid state (water), or gas state (vapor) for therapeutic purposes; the greater the difference in temperature between the body and the application, the greater the effect; the use of hydrotherapy can be categorized by its effect on the body

 1. Thermal
    a) Conduction—heat/cold pack on the body, hot/cold bath
    b) Convection—using a sauna
    c) Conversion—using ultrasound
 2. Mechanical—sprays, whirlpools
 3. Chemical—ingestion of water by mouth or irrigation

B. Cryotherapy (ice therapy)

 1. Local effects—short application will stimulate, long application will sedate
    a) Vasoconstriction (blood vessels get smaller)
    b) Decreases circulation to the area
 2. Systemic effects—short application will stimulate, long application will sedate
    a) The application of ice will cause the heart rate to increase to try and pump blood to the cold areas and therefore raise the metabolism
 3. Additional information on ice application
    a) Three stages of sensation for ice massage: burning, aching, and numbing; always work in the numb stage
    b) Penetrates the deepest into the tissue, therefore use when working deep
    c) Use ice on acute injuries; 20 minutes on, 20 minutes off
    d) Do not use ice on clients with Raynaud's or other impaired circulatory disorders
    e) Cold water is classified as 50–65°F
    f) Caution is used not to damage tissue through prolonged application
    g) The universal treatment for strains and sprains is RICE—Rest, Ice, Compression, and Elevation

C. Heat application

 1. Local effects of heat
    a) Vasodilation
    b) Increases circulation to the area
    c) Increases sweating
 2. Systemic effects of heat
    a) The application of heat will cause the heart rate to increase by trying to pump blood back toward the heart and therefore raise metabolism
    b) Increases the release of digestive juices and therefore the process of digestion

3. Additional information on heat application
   a) Use on chronic injuries
   b) Good for cramps/spasms
   c) Good for relaxation of soft tissues (muscles, tendons, ligaments) to improve pliability (stretching or ROM)
   d) Never apply heat to an inflamed area
   e) *Fomentation* is another name for a heat pack
   f) Moist heat penetrates deeper than dry
   g) Do not use on clients who have diminished sensation
   h) Do not use on clients with vascular disease
   i) Do not use on areas of hemorrhage
   j) Do not use on clients with cancer
   k) Hot water is classified as 100–115°F
   l) Caution is used not to burn the skin
   m) Temperatures used in a bath should not exceed 115°F
   n) Tepid water is categorized as 80–95°F
4. Additional information on hydrotherapy
   a) Contrast application of hot and cold is most effective in treating chronic disorder; always end the rotation with cold
   b) Hubbard tank uses a turbine for underwater exercise
   c) Baths include whirlpool, sitz (used to treat the pelvic/urogenital area), Russian (steam)
   d) Heliotherapy—light therapy

IV. PARAFFIN (HEATED WAX) TREATMENTS

A. Paraffin is used for both relaxation and medicinal purposes

B. Used over joints, on the hands, feet, old breaks, arthritis, and bursitis (in the sub-acute/chronic stage)

C. Never use paraffin over joint replacement or over the heart

D. Will make skin soft and moist prior to massage

V. ADJUNCT THERAPIES

A. Stretching

1. *Static*—stretch is held without movement
2. *Ballistic*—bouncing; NEVER recommended because it can create micro-tears in the soft tissue
3. *Range of motion* (*ROM*)—movement of a joint from one extreme of the articulation to the other; also called joint movements
   a) *Active*—the client moves into the stretched position unassisted by the MT
   b) *Passive*—the MT moves the client into a stretched position unassisted by client
   c) *Active assisted*—the MT and client work together to get to the desired stretched position
   d) *Active resistive*—the client actively moves a joint while the therapist applies resistance to the movement

4. When you want to determine if you have joint or ligament pain, you would passively move the joint through it's full ROM; this will disengage the muscles; if there is still pain, it is articular in nature

5. Isometric contraction of a muscle reeducates and resets the proprioceptors

B. **Muscle Energy Technique (MET)/Proprioceptive Neuromuscular Facilitation (PNF)**

1. *Contract-relax* (post-isometric relaxation)—after a muscle contracts, it relaxes (have client contract the hamstrings against resistance for 5–10 seconds; have client relax while you passively stretch the hamstrings until you meet resistance; slightly release the stretch and have client contract the hamstrings against resistance again; after each contraction the hamstrings can be stretched further because of post-isometric relaxation)

2. *Antagonist-contract* (reciprocal inhibition)—when a muscle contracts, the antagonist is automatically relaxed (to stretch the hamstrings (for knee flexion), position the leg so the hamstrings are stretched to slight resistance; have client contract the quadriceps against resistance for 5–10 seconds; have client relax and you passively stretch the hamstrings until you meet resistance; slightly release stretch and have client contract the quadriceps against resistance again; by contracting the quadriceps, the hamstrings are automatically relaxed and can be stretched further; used for spasms and cramps)

3. *Contract-relax-antagonist-contract* (CRAC)—combines post-isometric relaxation and reciprocal inhibition (to stretch the hamstrings (for hip extension), position the leg so the hamstrings are stretched to slight resistance; have client contract the hamstrings against resistance (isometric) then relax the hamstrings and contract the psoas (antagonist) against resistance; flexion of the hip will automatically stretch the hamstrings)

4. All of these techniques are used to improve ROM

C. **Myofascial techniques**

1. Address the fascial system of the body; when fascia becomes tight and restricted, it causes limitations in mobility, abnormal postural deviations, and pain; by addressing the fascial restrictions in the body, the client will experience relief from these symptoms

   a) *Bindegewebsmassage* (connective tissue massage)—developed by Elizabeth Dicke; believed to relieve restrictions in fascia therefore improving circulation in the connective tissue and ultimately the internal organs

      (1) Cross-fiber or transverse friction are considered part of connective tissue massage; used to treat sub-acute injuries, and to break up adhesions in the tissue

      (2) Dr. James Cyriax developed Deep Transverse Friction Massage

  b) *Rolfing* (structural integration)—developed by Dr. Ida Rolf; attempts to align the body around the vertical axis through manipulation of the myofascial tissue; 10 treatments

  c) *Myofascial release/unwinding*—developed by John Barnes; slow, intentional stretching of the myofascial system

   (1) Uses little to no lotion

   (2) Can be incorporated into a full body Swedish massage

   (3) When there are adhesions in the myofascial system, there would be a decrease in muscular movement and an increase in risk of injury

D. Passive positioning

1. The least invasive of the soft tissue manipulation therapies; there are three categories: strain-counterstrain, orthobionomy, and structural muscular balancing

  a) *Strain-counterstrain*—developed by Dr. Lawrence Jones; press down on tender points located in the affected tissue; move client into a position of maximum comfort and the pain in the tender points will disappear; hold that position for 90 seconds, then slowly bring client back to neutral position

  b) *Orthobionomy*—developed by Dr. Arthur Pauls; composed of both physical and energy methods; move client into comfortable position and support them there; uses trigger point and passive joint movement to alleviate pain and discomfort

  c) *Structural/muscular balancing*—developed by Dr. Ray Lichtman; also known as positional release; bring client into a state of comfort, gently compress into the joint for 30–90 seconds, and passively return to neutral

E. Craniosacral therapy

1. Developed by William Sutherland and John Upledger

2. Subtle bodywork that affects the autonomic nervous system; practitioner attempts to "feel" the craniosacral rhythm; involves the movement of the craniosacral fluid through the dural tube; 6–12 cycles per minute; therapist attempts to achieve "still points"; there are many holds including placing one hand on the sacrum and the other on the cranium; used to treat many ailments including autism in children

F. Manual lymph drainage

1. Developed by Dr. Emil Vodder

2. Consists of slow, light, rhythmic strokes that assist in the return of lymph from the interstitial spaces to the circulatory system; used to remove excess fluid from the tissues, improve healing and treat lymphatic disorders

G. Feldenkrais

1. Founded by Dr. Moshe Feldenkrais

2. The Feldenkrais Method consists of slow, gentle body movement and awareness through imaging; this is a 1-1 method that works to

have the client feel the quality of change in their body; it can improve relaxation, flexibility, and coordination

H. Hellerwork
1. Founded by Joseph Heller
2. Hellerwork is a combination of connective tissue and gentle deep tissue massage, movement, and dialogue; this method works on the belief that everyone is innately healthy and that through reeducation in 11 sessions, one can reconnect the body, mind, and spirit for optimal balance in the body

I. Trager
1. Founded by Dr. Milton Trager
2. Consists of light, rhythmical rocking and shaking of the body that will help loosen joints, relieve tension, and improve flexibility; "hook-up" is the state of awareness the practitioner is in while giving the 60–90 minute session; mentastics are exercises done mentally by the client after the session to maintain the successes of the treatment

J. Reflexology
1. Developed by Dr. William Fitzgerald
2. Based on the belief that the zones of the body are directly related to points on the hands, feet, and ears; by stimulating the specified points, the therapist can reflexively affect the targeted body part

K. Neuromuscular therapy
1. Developed by Dr. Stanley Leif
2. Utilizes skin rolling, stretching, deep gliding, and direct compression to alleviate pain and dysfunction

L. Sport therapy
1. *Pre-event*—fast paced, invigorating massage to warm tissue and improve circulation
2. *Post-event*—slow, rhythmical massage given to restore the athlete's natural balance; removes metabolic waste, encourages pre-event circulation, and aids in muscle soreness; this is not a deep massage
3. *Rehabilitative/intercompetition massage*—done between events to address specific muscle soreness and injury prevention

M. Trigger point therapy
1. Developed by Dr. Janet Travell and David Simons
2. A point of hyperirritability that will cause pain, tenderness, and possibly referred pain; both active and latent trigger points cause dysfunction, but only active trigger points cause pain; referred pain does not follow dermatomes
   a) Referred pain from the subscapularis is concentrated in the posterior deltoid and may extend medially over the scapula, down the posterior aspect of the area and skip to a band across the waist
   b) Referred pain from the deltoid is concentrated locally in the anterior, middle, and posterior deltoid

N. Pregnancy massage

1. *First trimester*—no abdominal massage; client can comfortably lie in all positions; no deep massage in legs, reflexology, shiatsu, acupressure (especially reproductive points); risk of miscarriage is highest, therefore proceed with caution (especially when using aromatherapy)
2. *Second trimester*—bolster client under right hip to alleviate pressure on the inferior vena cava; no deep massage in legs, reflexology, shiatsu, acupressure (especially reproductive points); side-lying or semi-reclining position after 22 weeks; pillow/bolster between legs, under head, and under arm
3. *Third trimester*—side-lying or semi-reclining position only; no deep massage in legs, reflexology, shiatsu, or acupressure (especially reproductive points)
4. The side-lying position is also very useful when working with obese patients or those with respiratory disorders where lying supine is uncomfortable

VI. ENERGY THERAPIES

A. Reiki—developed by Dr. Mikao Usui; either gentle contact or no contact with the client; spiritual in nature; focuses on chi and clearing the chakras

B. Polarity—developed by Randolph Stone; includes life energy, chakras, and elements
1. *Elements*—earth, water, fire, air, and ether (descending to ascending)
   a) None of the other elements can occur without the ether element being open
   b) Ether is the only element that is different when compared to oriental
2. *Chakras* (energy centers)—root (red), sacral (orange), solar plexus (yellow), heart (green), throat (blue), third eye (indigo), crown (violet)
3. Gunas are the three principles of energy movement: tamas, rajas, and sattva; the exam may ask for the three gunas as the "types/depth of touch": Satvic, Rajas, and Tamas

C. Therapeutic touch—also known as "laying-on of hands"; has been used for many years by professional nursing organizations to promote balancing and healing of clients; it is a noninvasive treatment approach that addresses the individual physically, mentally, emotionally, and spiritually

VII. EASTERN THERAPIES

A. Eastern medicine treats the body as a whole—the spirit, physical and mental well being of the client is taken into consideration; the initial diagnosis of a client may include questioning, observing, listening/smelling, and touching; may include color of tongue and tongue "hair"; the most familiar Eastern therapies are listed here with country of origin

1. *Amma/anma*—ancient Japanese
2. *Acupuncture*—ancient Chinese
3. *Acupressure*—Western adaptation of acupuncture
4. *Thai*—Thailand
5. *Ayurvedic*—India
6. *Tui-na*—modern Chinese massage
7. *Shiatsu*—modern Japanese massage; literally means "finger pressure"
8. *Jin Shin Do*—modern acupressure/acupuncture; involves yoga, Taoism

B. **Below are some basic definitions to help the student better understand the following section**

1. *Life force*—can be known as chi, ki, qi, prana; chi is the energy that flows throughout the body
   a) Energy flows from superior to inferior and inferior to superior
   b) Disease occurs when there is an imbalance in chi
2. *Jitsu*—defined as an excess of chi
3. *Kyo*—defined as deficient chi
4. *Hara*—defined as the center of gravity/point of balance; located four finger-widths below the umbilicus deep in abdomen
5. *Tsubo*—points along the meridians
6. *Tsun/cun/sun*—width of the client's thumb; a unit of measurement
7. *Tao*—"the way"; made up of two opposite yet complimentary forces: yin and yang; one can not exist without the other
   a) *Chi* is the connection between yin and yang
   b) *Characteristics of Yin*—feminine, dark, cold, blood, body fluids, tissues, descending energy, passive, earth, interior
   c) *Characteristics of Yang*—masculine, light, heat, energy, ascending energy, day, mind, active, heaven, exterior
   d) If you think of yin and yang in terms of a mountain, the side that faces the sun is yang and the side shaded by the mountain is yin
   e) Yin energy flows from the earth toward the heavens
   f) Yang energy flows from the heavens toward the earth

C. **The Eastern therapies are all based on an internal energy system consisting of 12 meridians (six paired) and 2 extraordinary vessels; chi flows through these interconnected channels and if it becomes blocked, there is disease**

D. **There are five elements and six paired *meridians:* fire which contains two paired meridians (*heart/small intestine* and *pericardium/triple heater*); earth: one paired meridian (*stomach/spleen*); metal: one paired meridian (*lung/large intestine*); water: one paired meridian (*bladder/kidney*); and wood: one paired meridian (*gall bladder/liver*); the extraordinary vessels are the governing vessel and conception vessel**

E. Meridians

1. Meridians are "channels" that energy travels through all around the body; these lines are invisible and interconnected; there are superficial meridians and deep meridians
   a) Three yin meridians begin in the feet and terminate in the chest: spleen (Sp), liver (Li) and kidney (K)
   b) Three yin meridians begin in the chest and terminate in the fingertips: lung (Lu), pericardium (P) and heart (H)
   c) Yin meridians are located on the anterior and medial aspects of the body
   d) Three yang meridians begin in the fingertips and terminate in the face: large intestine (LI), small intestine (SI), and triple warmer (TW)
   e) Three yang meridians begin in the face and terminate in the feet: stomach (St), bladder (Bl), and gallbladder (GB)
   f) Yang meridians are located on the back or lateral aspects of the body; *except* Stomach; it is the only yang meridian on the front of the body
   g) The two meridians not associated with an organ are pericardium and triple warmer; they are referred to as supplemental fire
   h) Leg meridians (Yin) (lateral to medial): Sp, Li, K
   i) Leg meridians (Yang) (medial to lateral): Bl, GB, St
      (1) Remember these by using SiLK (i for yin), BaGS (a for yang)
   j) Arm meridians (Yin) (medial to lateral): Lu, P, H (LiPH)
   k) Arm meridians (Yang) (medial to lateral): LI, TH, SI (LaTS)
   l) The meridians listed below are in sequential order of the times that they are most active
2. Metal—Lung (L) (Yin), Large Intestine (LI) (Yang)
   a) L (11 points)—L1 begins on the coracoid process and travels up the radial side of the arm and ends on the radial side of the thumb; 3–5 a.m.
      (1) Chest pain
   b) LI (20 points)—LI1 begins on the radial side of the index finger and travels down the posterior radial side of the arm to the lateral corner of the nostril; 5–7 a.m.
      (1) Tennis elbow
      (2) Diverticulitis
3. Earth—Stomach (St) (Yang), Spleen (Sp) (Yin)
   a) St (45 points)—St1 begins below the center of the eyeball, travels down the anteriolateral aspect of the body and ends on the lateral side of the 2nd toe; 7–9 a.m.
      (1) Only yang meridian on the anterior body
   b) Sp (21 points)—Sp1 begins on the medial side of the big toe and travels up the anteriomedial aspect of the body into the armpit and ends on the 6th intercostal space; 9–11 a.m.
      (1) Governs/regulates blood
      (2) Sp4 and Sp6 are contraindicated for pregnancy

4. Fire—Heart (H) (Yin), Small Intestine (SI) (Yang)
    a) Heart (9 points)—H1 is in the armpit; the meridian travels across the medial aspect of the arm to the radial posterior corner of little finger; 11 a.m.–1 p.m.
        (1) Chest pain/palpitations
        (2) Creativity/mental faculties
    b) SI (19 points)—SI1 begins on the ULNAR posterior corner of the little finger, travels through the triceps around the shoulder to the TMJ; 1–3 p.m.
        (1) Neck and shoulder pain
        (2) Separates pure from impure
5. Water—Bladder (Bl) (Yang), Kidney (K) (Yin)
    a) Bl (67 points)—Bl1 begins on the medial corner of the eye and travels up over the head to the occiput where it splits in two; the two lines run parallel to each other through the erectors, gluteals and posterior thigh where they join again behind the knee (Bl 40); the meridian continues down the posterior leg to the lateral side of the little toe; 3–5 p.m.
        (1) Bl 23—Low back pain, edema, impotence
        (2) Regulates ANS
        (3) Sometimes referred to as the urinary bladder (UB)
    b) K (27 points)—K1 begins on the plantar surface of the foot and travels up the medial aspect of the leg and chest to the sternoclavicular joint; 5–7 p.m.
        (1) K3 contraindicated in pregnancy
        (2) Hypertension
        (3) Root of all yin
        (4) Osteoporosis
6. Supplemental fire—Pericardium (P) or Heart Constrictor (HC) (Yin) and Triple heater or triple warmer or triple burner (TH/TW/TB) (Yang)
    a) P (9 points)—P1 begins on the lateral side of the nipple and travels up the center of the arm to the radial side of the middle finger; 7–9 p.m.
        (1) Regulates the heart
        (2) Chest pain
    b) TH (23 points)—TH1 begins on the ulnar side of the ring finger, travels down through the extensors of the forearm, triceps, posterior deltoid, and trapezius around the ear to the lateral corner of the eyebrow; 9–11p.m.
        (1) Tinnitus
        (2) Migraines (TH5)
        (3) Headache (TH3, TH5)
        (4) Regulates lymphatic system
7. Wood—Gallbladder (GB) (Yang), Liver (L) (Yin)
    a) GB (44 points)—GB1 begins on the lateral corner of the eye, zigzags around the ear and head, down the lateral aspect of the

body and terminates on the lateral side of the 4th toe; 11 p.m.–1 a.m.

b) L (14 points)—L1 begins on the lateral side of the big toe, up the medial aspect of the leg and abdomen and ends directly under the nipple; 1 a.m.–3 a.m.

8. Conception vessel (CV; 24 points)—Begins in the perineum and travels straight up the anterior mid-sagittal line to the center of the bottom (inferior edge) of the lower lip
   a) Regulates all Yin meridians, functions, and energy
   b) Chi reserve for all Yin energy

9. Governing vessel (GV; 27 points)—Begins in the perineum and travels straight up the posterior mid-sagittal line to the center (superior edge) of the upper lip
   a) Regulates all Yang meridians, functions and energy
   b) Chi reserve for all Yang energy
   c) GV4—low back pain, impotence, edema

10. Additional information
   a) Contraindicated during pregnancy—LI4, Sp6, K3, GB21, CV4
   b) Headache points—Lu10, LI4, H3, GB20, L3, GV20
   c) Any question having to do with the back—answer is bladder
   d) Any question having to do with the lateral aspect or running along the coronal/frontal plane—answer is gallbladder
   e) Upper burner refers to the cardiovascular system
   f) Functions are summarized in the chart below:

Element	Fire	Earth	Metal	Water	Wood
Yin	Heart; Pericardium	Spleen	Lung	Kidney	Liver
Yang	Small intestine Triple warmer	Stomach	Large intestine	Bladder	Gallbladder
Function	Circulation	Digestion	Intake of chi (Lu); Elimination (LI)	Purification	Detoxification of chi, storage
Color	Red	Yellow	White	Blue, black	Green
Expression	Laughing	Singing	Weeping	Groaning	Shouting
Season	Summer	Indian summer	Fall	Winter	Spring
Sense	Speech	Taste	Smell	Hearing	Sight
Emotion	Shock	Worry	Grief	Fear	Anger
Body Tissue	Blood, BV	Flesh	Skin	Bones	Muscles
Taste	Bitter, burned	Sweet	Spicy	Salty	Sour
Times	H-11am–1pm SI-1–3pm P-7–9pm TW-9–11pm	St-7–9am Sp-9–11am	Lu-3–5am LI-5–7am	Bl-3–5pm K-5–7pm	GB-11pm–1am Li-1–3am

F. Cycles

1. *Generating (sheng)*—This cycle is creative; a saying to help remember: For Every Mother Was Woman
   a) *Fire* creates ashes and therefore earth, *earth* is made up of metals, *metal* transports water, *water* feeds wood, and *wood* feeds fire
   b) Questions regarding mother, grandmother, daughter, and so on will be answered with this cycle; i. e., what is the grandmother of fire? Find fire and go back two elements: Wood would be the mother and water is the grandmother
2. *Controlling (ko)*—this cycle allows for the control of one element by another; a saying to help remember: Watering Fires Makes Wood Embers
   a) *Water* controls fire by putting it out, *fire* controls metal by melting it, *metal* controls wood by cutting it, *wood* controls earth by covering it, and *earth* controls water by damming it
   b) The questions regarding the controlling cycle will be straightforward; they may ask what controls kidney? You would have two choices, stomach or spleen; the best answer would be stomach because it is the next meridian that the chi will flow to; but, if the choice were spleen, that would be the answer

VIII. BUSINESS PRACTICES

A. Ethics and professionalism—many questions will be asked on the examination pertaining to ethics and professionalism; when answering these questions, use common sense; be familiar with the laws pertaining to your state and if you are taking the NCBTMB examination, learn their Code of Ethics; the information below is just a guideline; it is assumed that your massage training included a thorough curriculum of ethics and professionalism
   1. The first and foremost rule of massage is: Do no harm
   2. Practice truth in advertising; never claim to be able to do anything that you cannot
   3. Begin screening your appointments with the first phone call; if a person calls and is interested in something other than therapeutic massage, you may be able to pick up on it in the initial contact
   4. Explain your fee scale, client expectations, and therapist expectations before the massage
   5. Educate yourself and your clients about the therapeutic value of massage
   6. Remember to tell the client both positive and negative effects the massage may have on his or her body
   7. Greet your clients by standing up and shaking their hand etc.; be warm and welcoming; try to convey to your client that they are in a safe, friendly, and therapeutic environment
   8. Remember that first impressions go a long way

9. Always ask your clients if this is their first massage before proceeding with anything; explain what they can expect, that they will need to disrobe to their level of comfort, how you would like them positioned on the table, how you perform your routine, etc.; this will help to calm the anxieties the client is experiencing; it will make the MT appear to be much more professional and caring as well

10. Be cautious about where you distribute business cards

11. It is always nice to give back to your community; if you can afford to do a little pro bono work, you should

12. Educate the public on the effects and benefits of therapeutic massage whenever possible; give a free seminar/demonstration etc.

13. Take continuing education classes—no one knows it all

14. Do not perform any activity outside your scope of practice

15. Refer clients to proper professionals when necessary

16. Do not date clients

17. Do not do "favors" for clients that are illegal or immoral

18. Adhere to local and state laws

19. Do not partake in any sexual activity with clients

20. Stop any sexual advances immediately; *silence is acceptance*

21. Keep detailed medical history assessments and update regularly

22. If a client refuses to fill out a medical questionnaire, verbally ask the client the information

23. Never perform a massage without the information you need to provide a safe and effective massage

24. Encourage client to contact physician if you find a pathology of which the client was not aware

25. MT's attire should be appropriate; not too tight, too loose, too see-through or gaudy

26. Do not wear jewelry, T-shirts, or hats that may offend

27. Jewelry should be kept simple and not too long as to interfere with the massage

28. Never attempt to diagnose, prescribe or let your client believe that you know more than their physician or a more highly trained professional

IX. RECORD KEEPING

A. Record keeping is one of the most important practices for running a successful business; the questions pertaining to record keeping are going to be geared toward your understanding of filing tax returns, what forms you need to fill out, write-offs, and your knowledge of SOAP charting, medical history checklists and intake forms. Again, this information is only a general guideline, you should consult a professional to answer any questions of which you are not sure

1. Each client should fill out an initial intake form, a medical history checklist, and possibly an "agreement" stating what the client can

expect from you and what you expect from the client; these forms should be updated every 6 months

2. Keep all records confidential; do not leave them open on counters where others will have a chance to read them

3. Keep SOAP notes (Subjective, Objective, Assessment, and Progress) on each client; you will want to refer to them before each visit with your client; SOAP charting is a necessity when you are working with insurance companies

4. Bill insurance companies honestly; do not do or accept "favors"

5. Never release medical records without a signed release of information form

6. Report 100% of your cash earnings to the IRS

7. You must report all barter income to the IRS

8. Keep records of treatment and progress to better treat your clients

9. If you are self-employed (independent contractor), you must file a form 1099 to the IRS; you will be responsible for paying your own taxes; you should keep meticulous records for write-offs including equipment, supplies, travel etc.; you will fill out a Schedule C for these deductions; you will also be required to file estimated tax returns quarterly (1040 ES); you should hire an accountant to help you with these issues

10. If another person employs you, they will provide you with a salary; your employer is responsible for paying your taxes and you will file a W-2 at the end of the year

11. As a sole-proprietor (you have an actual place of business), you will file a Schedule C, and pay your own taxes that you file at the end of the year

12. If you are in a partnership, you will file a Schedule K and Form 1065

13. Malpractice insurance is not a requirement for MTs, however when you join professional organizations (AMTA, ABMP, etc.), you have the option of buying insurance through the organization

14. Liability and property damage insurance is required for a massage establishment

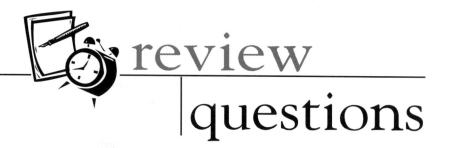

DIRECTIONS Each of the questions or incomplete statements below is followed by suggested answers or completions. Select the one answer that is best in each case.

1. Fear is associated with which element?
   A. Water
   B. Wood
   C. Earth
   D. Fire

2. You have left a chart open on the counter. What ethical code are you violating?
   A. Liability
   B. Scope of practice
   C. Confidentiality
   D. SOAP

3. You are working on a client who was recently involved in an MVA (motor vehicle accident) and the client would like you to add ten more treatments on to settle the claim. What should you do?
   A. Call the insurance adjuster
   B. Report your client for fraud
   C. Call either attorney
   D. Advise your client to speak with their attorney to get more treatment for the injury

4. What is the most important protocol for documenting progress of your client?
   A. RICE
   B. SOAP
   C. ANS
   D. TXS

5. What is the most important question you should ask a client you are seeing for the first time?
   A. Client history
   B. Emergency contact person
   C. Have you ever had a massage before?
   D. Are you currently taking any medication?

6. How much of a barter agreement do you have to claim to the IRS?
   A. 25%
   B. 50%
   C. 75%
   D. 100%

7. What type of insurance do MTs buy to cover their work in case a client sues?
   A. Malpractice
   B. Homeowner
   C. Life
   D. Liability

8. Which therapy includes acupuncture, acupressure, yoga, and Taoism?
   A. Jin Shin Do
   B. Reiki
   C. Feldenkrais
   D. Rolfing

9. Which chakra is represented by the color green?
   A. Throat
   B. Heart

82

C. Sacral

D. Crown

10. The therapy that is performed either with no contact or light contact with the body is:
    A. Craniosacral.
    B. Rolfing.
    C. Jin Shin Do.
    D. Reiki.

11. Which of the following are correctly paired meridians?
    A. Liver and Kidney
    B. Heart and Stomach
    C. Stomach and Spleen
    D. Stomach and Large Intestine

12. Massaging Sp4 is contraindicated for:
    A. Migraines.
    B. Fracture.
    C. Angina.
    D. Pregnancy.

13. In oriental medicine, how does energy flow?
    A. Up and down
    B. Forward and back
    C. Anterior and posterior
    D. Contralateral

14. In draping during massage, you always cover the:
    A. Chest.
    B. Stomach.
    C. Pelvic area.
    D. Legs.

15. Which meridian has its endpoint on the little toe?
    A. GB
    B. Bl
    C. H
    D. Sp

16. A client came in for massage and requested to be massaged on the back only. You would do the following?
    A. Massage the client as requested.
    B. Tell the client that you always massage the whole body because it feels good.
    C. Tell the client to come back when she is ready for a full body massage.
    D. Tell the client okay, and massage the whole body.

17. Chi in oriental medicine means:
    A. Energy lines.
    B. The center.
    C. Life force.
    D. Control.

18. Which form do you have to file if you have a business partner?
    A. Schedule K
    B. 1040 EZ
    C. Schedule D
    D. 1040 SL

19. When do you release a client's medical record?
    A. When the insurance company requests a copy of the record.
    B. When the attorney calls for it.
    C. When the client calls you one the phone and requests it.
    D. When the client signs a release of information form.

20. If a client requests an energy massage, whom would you refer them to?
    A. Polarity therapist
    B. NMT
    C. Reflexologist
    D. Rolfer

21. What is the main purpose of performing post-event massage?
    A. Stimulate the muscles
    B. Reduce swelling in sprains/strains
    C. Rid the body of metabolic waste build-up
    D. Treat adhesions

22. A client has scar tissue on the TFL. Which of the following would be the best massage treatment?
    A. Tapotement
    B. Friction
    C. Vibration
    D. Petrissage

23. What is the correct order for SOAP charting?
    A. Support, Objective, Active, Passive
    B. Stretching, Observation, Active, Passive
    C. Subjective, Objective, Assessment, Planning
    D. Sight, Olfactory, Auditory, Progress

24. When performing polarity therapy:
    A. The mind and body are treated separately.
    B. The mind and body are treated together.
    C. The mind is treated, not the body.
    D. The body is treated, not the mind.

25. Rolfing is a form of:
    A. Connective tissue massage.
    B. Energy work.
    C. ROM.
    D. Vascular disease.

26. What type of oil would you use if you did not want to stain your linens?
    A. Rosewater oil
    B. Cold-pressed oil
    C. Water-dispersible oil
    D. Mineral oil

27. Why would you ask a client if they would like music playing during their massage?
    A. To see if they are hearing impaired
    B. To see if they are paying attention to what you say
    C. To see if they are mentally impaired
    D. To see if they would like a quiet massage environment

28. A female client reports her husband has recently passed away. Which of the following actions is appropriate?
    A. Prescribe an antidepressant.
    B. Be empathetic, adjust the massage accordingly, and watch for her response.
    C. Give her psychotherapy.
    D. Tell her it will be okay.

29. The rate of the craniosacral rhythm is defined as:
    A. 6–12 beats/minute.
    B. 12–15 beats/minute.
    C. 15–20 beats/minute.
    D. 18–21 beats/minute.

30. In which position would you massage a pregnant client in that was in her third trimester?
    A. Inverted
    B. Prone
    C. Side-lying
    D. Massage in the third trimester is contraindicated

31. The meridian which zigzags around the head and travels down the lateral side of the body ends on the:
    A. Little toe.
    B. Little finger.
    C. Fourth toe.
    D. Fourth finger.

32. Where does the conception vessel begin?
    A. Superior aspect of upper lip
    B. Inferior aspect of lower lip
    C. Perineum
    D. Proximal to the umbilicus

33. A client presents with extremely thin, brittle hair, and dark circles under the eyes. What should you do?
    A. Encourage client to call her physician.
    B. Do a stimulating massage.
    C. Prescribe nutrients.
    D. Refer to psychologist.

34. As you walk into the waiting area, your next client is looking you up and down. What should you do?
    A. Tell the client that you are not going to be able to do the massage.

B. Explain the massage procedure and expectations of client and therapist.

C. Ignore it, it will stop.

D. Get your fee up front in case you have to stop the massage early.

35. For which of the following chronic pathologies would you not apply a hot pack?
A. Ankylosing spondylitis
B. Osteoarthritis
C. Edema
D. Rheumatoid arthritis

36. The popliteal area is an endangerment site for which structure?
A. Femoral nerve
B. Tibial nerve
C. Jugular artery
D. Carotid artery

37. While pressing on a tender point in the deltoids, the client reports feeling pain in another area of the body. What is this called?
A. Phantom pain
B. Cramp
C. Sprain
D. Referred pain

38. You place one hand on the sacrum and one on the base of the cranium. Which system is affected?
A. Skeletal
B. Respiratory
C. Digestive
D. Lymphatic

39. A client liked your massage so much that she told you to go ahead and bill the insurance company for massage not given. What do you do?
A. Inform the insurance company.
B. Call the police.
C. Inform the client that it would be illegal to do that.
D. Do as the client requested.

40. Which meridian would you work for a client that complains of heart palpitations?

A. GB
B. CV
C. Bl
D. H

41. A runner comes to the massage tent after a race and complains of a hamstring spasm. What muscle needs to be stretched?
A. Hamstring
B. Gastrocnemius
C. Quadriceps
D. Tibialis anterior

42. The time associated with the Stomach meridian is:
A. 3–5 a.m.
B. 5–7 a.m.
C. 7–9 a.m.
D. 9–11 a.m.

43. In which endangerment site is the carotid artery found?
A. Anterior triangle of the neck
B. Posterior triangle of the neck
C. Femoral triangle
D. Posterior femoral triangle

44. What are the chakras?
A. Energy pathways
B. Energy channels
C. Energy centers
D. Channel pathways

45. In Sanskrit, what does "guna" mean?
A. Principles of motion/movement
B. Principles of kinesiology
C. Principles of physiology/pathology
D. Principles of body/mind connection

46. A trigger point is defined as:
A. A hypoirritable spot in the soft tissue that can cause pain and referred pain.
B. A hyperirritable spot in the soft tissue that can cause pain and referred pain.
C. The endpoint of joint mobilization.
D. The endpoint for CRAC technique.

47. This stroke is used to begin and end the massage:
    A. Petrissage.
    B. Effleurage.
    C. Friction.
    D. Vibration.

48. Which stroke would be used to treat adhesions/scar tissue?
    A. Petrissage
    B. Effleurage
    C. Friction
    D. Vibration

49. The gunas are:
    A. Tamas, rajas, slava.
    B. Rajas, prana, tasla.
    C. Kana, ramna, dana.
    D. Sattva, rajas, tamas.

50. Which meridian would you work to treat: low back pain, edema, and impotence?
    A. Sp
    B. Bl
    C. GB
    D. K

51. A client with fibromyalgia would benefit most from application of:
    A. Ice.
    B. Fomentation.
    C. Contrast bath.
    D. Heliotherapy.

52. These meridians make up the metal element:
    A. Heart/Lung.
    B. Lung/Small Intestine.
    C. Large Intestine/Heart.
    D. Lung/Large Intestine.

53. The GV regulates all:
    A. Yang.
    B. Yin.
    C. Tao.
    D. Chi.

54. The CV regulates all:
    A. Yang.
    B. Yin.
    C. Tao.
    D. Chi.

55. A client complains of back pain. Which meridian would you work?
    A. GB
    B. Lu
    C. UB
    D. CV

56. The elements associated with polarity therapy are:
    A. Fire, Earth, Metal, Water, Ether.
    B. Fire, Earth, Metal, Water, Wind.
    C. Fire, Earth, Metal, Water, Wood.
    D. Fire, Earth, Metal, Water, Stone.

57. LI4, LI10, LI20 would be worked to treat:
    A. Low back pain.
    B. Shoulder/neck pain.
    C. Lateral leg pain.
    D. Chest pain.

58. The oriental therapy that literally means "finger pressure" is:
    A. Jin Shin Do.
    B. Acupressure.
    C. Shiatsu.
    D. Acupuncture.

59. Yin energy flows:
    A. From inferior to superior.
    B. From superior to inferior.
    C. From lateral to medial.
    D. From Medial to lateral.

60. A client reports having dissociative disorder. How would you conduct the massage?
    A. Observe and adjust the massage accordingly.
    B. Counsel the client accordingly.
    C. Prescribe herbal supplements.
    D. Do not massage.

61. A client presents with a cramp in the hamstrings. What would be the best treatment?
    A. Deep effleurage on the hamstrings
    B. Deep transverse friction on the hamstrings
    C. Reciprocal inhibition with compression on the hamstrings
    D. Reciprocal inhibition with compression on the quadriceps

62. After a muscle contracts, it becomes inhibited and relaxes. This is best known as:
    A. CRAC.
    B. RICE.
    C. Antagonist contract.
    D. Tense-relax.

63. A client reports being abused as a child. What behavior might you expect?
    A. Inappropriate laughing
    B. Sexual inappropriateness
    C. Both a and b
    D. Neither a or b

64. A client presents with a sub-acute ankle sprain. What stroke would be most effective in treating the sprain?
    A. Vibration
    B. Friction
    C. Petrissage
    D. Tapotement

65. The best way for a client to get off the table after the massage is:
    A. Roll onto their side and slowly sit up.
    B. Rock back and forth until they sit up.
    C. Roll onto their back and drop one leg over the table.
    D. Rock from side to side until they reach the side of the table.

66. The most effective hydrotherapy treatment for chronic injuries is:
    A. Ice.
    B. Heat.
    C. Paraffin.
    D. Contrast application of cold/heat.

67. All of the following are types of tapotement except:
    A. Slapping.
    B. Tapping.
    C. Whacking.
    D. Rapping.

68. This strokes is used to assist in venous return and milk the tissue:
    A. Effleurage.   C. Friction.
    B. Petrissage.   D. Tapotement.

69. The most widely recognized benefit of massage is:
    A. Release of lactic acid build-up.
    B. Improved circulation and relaxation.
    C. Pain management and cancer control.
    D. Cellulite control and improved skin tone.

70. The proper stance for giving a massage is:
    A. Knees bent, shifting body weight from front to back foot, and elbows close to the body.
    B. Knees and elbows locked with arms outstretched.
    C. One foot perpendicular to the other with weight on the back foot.
    D. Feet parallel to the table with weight on the front foot.

71. The universal treatment for minor sprains and strains is:
    A. SOAP.   C. SITS.
    B. MET.   D. RICE.

72. A client refuses to fill out the intake and medical history form. You should:
    A. Refuse to do the massage until they fill out the forms.
    B. Do the massage and send the form home with the client and have him or her bring it back later.
    C. Ask the client questions during the massage.
    D. Ask the client questions while explaining the massage procedure.

review questions

73. During the massage, a client becomes sexually inappropriate. You should:
    A. Call the police.
    B. Tell the client that their behavior is inappropriate and continue the massage.
    C. Explain to the client their behavior is inappropriate and end the massage.
    D. Ignore it, it will probably go away on its own.

74. Hook-up and mentastics are terms associated with:
    A. Hellerwork.
    B. Trigger point therapy.
    C. Shiatsu.
    D. Traeger.

75. Your client is obese and has a hard time breathing in the supine position. What might you do?
    A. Place a pillow under her knees.
    B. Place a pillow under her low back.
    C. Place the client in the side-lying position.
    D. Place the client in the prone position.

76. The break down of adhesions/scar tissue and muscle relaxation are considered:
    A. Thermal effects of massage.
    B. Mechanical effects of massage.
    C. Chemical effects of massage.
    D. Psychological effects of massage.

77. The structure located in the lumbar region which makes it an endangerment site is:
    A. Sacrum.
    B. Coccyx.
    C. Kidney.
    D. Bladder.

78. In performing Western massage, gliding strokes are:
    A. Centripetal.
    B. Centrifugal.
    C. Retroperitoneal.
    D. Ipsilateral.

79. A client presents with edema in the ankles. The order of massage should be:
    A. Foot, ankle, leg, hip.
    B. Hip, leg, ankle, foot.
    C. Toes, foot, ankle, leg.
    D. Ankle, foot, toe, leg.

80. Relaxation, stress reduction, and improved well-being are examples of:
    A. Thermal effects of massage.
    B. Mechanical effects of massage.
    C. Chemical effects of massage.
    D. Psychological effects of massage.

81. The single most important means of stopping the spread of germs/infection is:
    A. Proper hand-washing.
    B. Taking a shower daily.
    C. Wearing clean clothes.
    D. Using bleach on floors and in bathrooms.

82. Massage disappeared during the:
    A. Renaissance.
    B. Middle Ages.
    C. Revolution.
    D. Depression.

83. The vascular response to the application of cryotherapy is:
    A. Vasoconstriction.
    B. Vasodilation.
    C. Thrombosis.
    D. Embolism.

84. The vascular response to the application of a fomentation is:
    A. Vasoconstriction.
    B. Vasodilation.
    C. Thrombosis.
    D. Embolism.

85. The application of heat is contraindicated for:
    A. Chronic muscle strain.
    B. Sub-acute muscle strain.
    C. Edema.
    D. Fibromyalgia.

86. An athlete just completed a rigorous athletic competition. She is not sweating, she is staggering, and is incoherent. These symptoms indicate:
    A. Heat cramps.
    B. Heat exhaustion.
    C. Heat stroke.
    D. Hypothermia.

87. During a soccer game, your athlete turned their ankle and heard a snap. The ankle is swollen and deformed. This indicates:
    A. Sprain.
    B. Strain.
    C. Cramp.
    D. Spasm.

88. During the massage, your client gets a cramp in her gastrocnemius. You should have her contract the:
    A. Gastrocnemius.
    B. Tibialis anterior.
    C. Tibialis posterior.
    D. Quadriceps.

89. In a medical emergency, the first thing you should do is:
    A. Check ABCs.
    B. Clear the area of potential hazards.
    C. Move victim to a safe area.
    D. Call 911.

90. Zone therapy and reflex points in the feet, hands or ears are associated with:
    A. Jin Shin Do.
    B. Rolfing.
    C. Reflexology.
    D. Hellerwork.

91. As an independent contractor, you are required to:
    A. File quarterly estimated taxes.
    B. Pay taxes at the end of the year.
    C. You don't have to pay taxes.
    D. File a Schedule K.

92. Truth in advertising is important for all of the following except:
    A. Referrals.
    B. Repeat business.
    C. Tax write-offs.
    D. Professional integrity.

93. As a partner in a massage business, you are required to file a:
    A. Schedule L.
    B. Schedule K.
    C. Schedule B.
    D. Schedule D.

94. A general contraindication for hydrotherapy is:
    A. Chronic muscle strain.
    B. Peripheral nerve damage.
    C. Sub-acute muscle sprain.
    D. Full bony union.

95. The massage stroke used over nerve trunks and centers is:
    A. Effleurage.
    B. Petrissage.
    C. Friction.
    D. Vibration.

96. When massaging the abdomen, it is best accessed by:
    A. Elevating the lower leg in the supine position.
    B. Bending the knees so the pelvis is flexed forward in the supine position.
    C. Elevating the head and arms in the supine position.
    D. Bending the knees and extending the hip in the prone position.

97. Connective tissue massage addresses:
    A. Adhesions/restrictions in the fascia.
    B. Trigger points and referred pain.
    C. Reflex points of the feet and hands.
    D. Psychological disorders.

98. Effleurage strokes are used to:
    A. Distribute lubricant and assess tissue.
    B. Milk the tissue of metabolic waste.
    C. Stimulate nerve receptors.
    D. Disrupt adhesions.

99. The object of pre-event massage is to:
    A. Stimulate circulation.
    B. Restore circulation.

C. Break up adhesions.
D. Sedate the athlete.

100. The first rule of massage:
    A. Collect fees before the massage.
    B. Do no harm.
    C. Never do a free massage.
    D. Always do what the client requests.

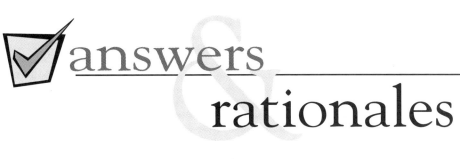

answers & rationales

The answer key will give you two pieces of information. The first is the correct answer, the second is the rationale.

1.
A. Review the table in the text

2.
C. All records should be put away where no one can read them

3.
D. Always abide by the law

4.
B. RICE is the universal treatment for sprains and strains

5.
C. Ask this first; then explain the massage, expectations for client and therapist, then review the intake form, etc.

6.
D. All income—cash, barter, charge, etc.—are required to be reported to the IRS

7.
A. Liability insurance is necessary for the establishment

8.
A. The other choices do not include yoga and Taoism

9.
B. Root (red), sacral (orange), solar plexus (yellow), heart (green), throat (blue), third eye (indigo), and crown (violet)

10.
D. One of the energy therapies

11.
C. They belong to the Earth element

12.
D. The spleen meridian travels through the abdomen

13.
A. Yin energy flows from the earth to the heavens, yang from the heavens to the earth

14.
C. The chest does not have to be draped on a male

15.
B. Review beginning and end points in the text

16.
A. Be flexible; this is your client's massage

17.
C. Chi is the energy of life

18.
A. Schedule K has to be filed for a partnership

19.
D. Medical records are to be released with client approval or a court order

20.
A. Polarity is one of the energy therapies

21.
C. Post-event massage is done to return the body to normal functioning

22.
B. Friction is used to treat adhesions and scar tissue

23.
C. This format is the common medical charting procedure

24.
B. There is no separation of mind and body in Polarity

25.
A. Restores normal body functioning around a vertical axis

26.
C. Water dispersible oils will wash out of your linens

27.
D. Not everyone wants to listen to music during the massage

28.
B. Always be aware of your client's response to the massage

29.
A. Review craniosacral therapy in the text

30.
C. Massage in the third trimester can be semi-reclining or side-lying

31.
C. 44 points in the GB meridian; remember: "44 in the 4th"

32.
C. Begins in the perineum and ends on the bottom of the lower lip

33.
A. Contact client's attending physician with any concerns

34.
B. Never leave any question in the client's mind that you perform therapeutic massage. *Silence is acceptance.*

35.
C. Never apply heat to an inflamed area

36.
B. The only nerve listed located in the posterior leg

37.
D. Referred pain arises from a TP but is felt in a different area

38.
B. Review craniosacral therapy in text

39.
C. Always abide by the law

40.
D. Review the heart meridian in the text

41.
A. Key word: stretched

42.
C. Review times of activity in the text

43.
A. Anterior triangle includes carotid, jugular arteries, and the vagus nerve

44.
C. Energy channels and pathways are meridians

45.
A. Review energy therapies section in text

46.
B. Review definition in text

47.
B. The most widely used stroke in massage

48.
C. The deepest stroke in massage

49.
D. Review energy therapies section in text

50.
B. Any question to do with the back; the answer is Bl

51.
B. Ice can intensify the pain

52.
D. Review meridians/elements in text

53.
A. Conception vessel regulates all yin

54.
B. Governing vessel regulates all yang

55.
C. UB (urinary bladder) is the same as Bl

56.
A. When you see ether, the answer is polarity

57.
B. The LI meridian travels along the posterior arm and through the shoulder

58.
C. Review definition of Shiatsu

59.
A. Yang energy flows superior to inferior

60.
A. Always be aware of your client's response to the massage

61.
C. Reciprocal inhibition is contraction of the opposing muscle/group and stretching the involved muscle/group

62.
D. After a muscle contracts, it will immediately relax

63.
C. Reactions to healthy touch may vary by client. Be aware of your client's response and adjust the massage accordingly

64.
B. Key word: sub-acute

65.
A. The other choices are dangerous

66.
D. Contrast therapy has been found to be the most effective treatment in treating chronic injuries

67.
C. Hacking, cupping, slapping, tapping, clapping, rapping, and pincement

68.
B. Key words: milk the tissue

69.
B. Key words: most widely recognized

70.
A. Proper body mechanics will avoid injury to therapist

71.
D. Universal treatment for sprains and strains

72.
D. You should not perform a massage without all the needed information

73.
C. Never leave any room for misunderstanding

74.
D. Key words: hook-up and mentastics

75.
C. Side-lying can be used for many different clients

76.
B. The manual manipulation of tissue is mechanical

77.
C. Located just below the rib cage on both sides of the body

78.
A. Centrifugal is away from point of reference

79.
B. Always clear the upper channels first when working with edema

80.
D. All have to do with the state of mind of the client

81.
A. Proper hand washing is imperative in stopping the spread of germs

82.
B. A time of repression of all the arts

83.
A. Vasodilation occurs with the application of heat

84.
B. Vasoconstriction occurs with the application of cold

85.
C. Never apply heat to an area of inflammation

86.
C. Refer to medical professionals immediately; life-threatening

87.
A. Key word: deformity

88.
B. By contracting the tibialis anterior, the gastrocnemius is stretched

89.
D. The first step is to ensure you have medical professionals on the way

90.
C. Reflex points in the feet, hands, and ears affect other parts of the body

91.
A. As an independent contractor you must file estimated quarterly taxes

92.
C. Tax write-offs have nothing to do with truth in advertising

93.
B. Schedule K has to be filed for a partnership

94.
B. Never use hydrotherapy with clients who experience impaired sensation

95.
D. Used as a sedating or stimulating stroke over nerve trunks/centers

96.
B. This position will relax the abdominal muscles for easier access

97.
A. Friction, cross-fiber friction, etc.

98.
A. Most widely used stroke in massage

99.
A. Pre-event massage is performed to prepare the athlete for competition

100.
B. Universal rule for massage

5 Practice Examination

contents

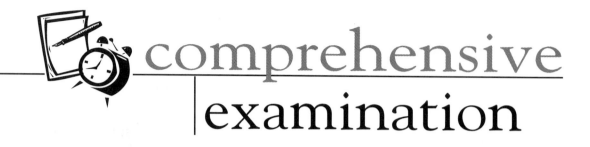

comprehensive examination

DIRECTIONS Each of the questions or incomplete statements below is followed by suggested answers or completions. Select the one answer that is best in each case.

---

1. Shin splints are a result of microtears of the:
   A. Extensor digitorum tendon.
   B. Flexor digitorum tendon.
   C. Periosteum around the tibia.
   D. Periosteum around the calcaneus.

2. Yang energy flows from:
   A. Superior to inferior.
   B. Inferior to superior.
   C. Posterior to anterior.
   D. Anterior to posterior.

3. Referred pain from a TP in the subscapularis may be felt in the:
   A. SCM.
   B. Biceps brachii.
   C. Pectoralis major.
   D. Waist.

4. Satvic, Rajas, and Tamas are:
   A. Types of touch.
   B. Chakras.
   C. Concentric contractions.
   D. Neuromuscular tests.

5. The term "Upper Burner" refers to the:
   A. Digestive system.
   B. Respiratory system.
   C. Integumentary system.
   D. Excretory system.

6. The purpose of post-event sport massage is:
   A. Stimulation of the athlete.
   B. Reduction in parasympathetic activity.
   C. Removal of metabolic waste build-up.
   D. Address injury through deep transverse friction and intense stretching.

7. A client reports having scoliosis. During the massage, you would concentrate on:
   A. Bilateral contraction of the spinal muscles.
   B. Unilateral contraction of the QL.
   C. Bilateral contraction of the TFL.
   D. Ipsilateral contraction of the levator scapula.

8. Referred pain from a TP in the posterior deltoid will be felt:
   A. Across the waist.
   B. In the SCM.
   C. Anteriorly in the pectoralis minor.
   D. Locally in the posterior deltoid.

9. A doctor writes a prescription for your client indicating "massage for comfort." This may mean that your client is:
   A. Post-operative.
   B. Terminally ill.
   C. Pre-operative.
   D. Menopausal.

10. Connective tissue massage may include:
    A. Transverse friction over tendons and ligaments.
    B. Holding static pressure on tsubos.
    C. Clearing the chakras.
    D. Both a and c.

11. Which of the following statements is true concerning pregnancy massage:
    A. Relaxation massage is always indicated.
    B. Rocking is indicated for the client experiencing morning sickness.
    C. Massage is contraindicated during pregnancy.
    D. Deep tissue massage on legs is indicated in all trimesters.

12. The stomach meridian is the only:
    A. Yin meridian on the anterior aspect of the body.
    B. Yin meridian on the posterior aspect of the body.
    C. Yang meridian on the anterior aspect of the body.
    D. Yang meridian on the posterior aspect of the body.

13. The relaxation response is activated by the:
    A. Sympathetic nervous system.
    B. Parasympathetic nervous system.
    C. Integumentary system.
    D. Digestive system.

14. Body position is controlled by the:
    A. Autonomic nervous system.
    B. Parasympathetic nervous system.
    C. Sympathetic nervous system
    D. Peripheral nervous system.

15. Deep pressure in the abdomen may endanger this structure:
    A. Radial nerve.
    B. Kidneys.
    C. Carotid artery.
    D. Aorta.

16. This meridian begins on the plantar surface of the foot:
    A. Kidney.
    B. Large intestine.
    C. Spleen.
    D. Stomach.

17. Which massage stroke is used to effect underlying structures by moving superficial layers of tissue over deep layers of tissue?
    A. Petrissage
    B. Effleurage
    C. Friction
    D. Tapotement

18. While performing passive ROM on a client, they report pain. You can safely assume that the injury/restriction involved is:
    A. Muscular.
    B. Ligamentous.
    C. Tendinous.
    D. Articular.

19. The Hara is considered the:
    A. Center of gravity.
    B. Way.
    C. "Upper burner."
    D. Pericardium.

20. An antagonist to the biceps brachii is:
    A. Brachioradialis.
    B. Triceps.
    C. Brachialis.
    D. Pectoralis minor.

21. A client reports having hurt her ankle yesterday. Upon examination, you find it is swollen and she can not move it. What should you do?
    A. Passive ROM
    B. Lymph drainage to eliminate the swelling
    C. Friction the tendons and ligaments
    D. Encourage client to contact her physician or visit the emergency room

22. Which massage stroke is most effective for post-fracture care?
    A. Friction
    B. Effleurage
    C. Vibration
    D. Petrissage

23. Too much insulin production is typical of:
    A. Type I diabetes.
    B. Type II diabetes.
    C. Leukemia.
    D. Anemia.

24. Lack of blood flow to an area is defined as:
    A. Hyperemia.
    B. Atrophy.
    C. Ischemia.
    D. Hypoxia.

25. There are three lobes in the:
    A. Left lung.
    B. Right lung.
    C. Left kidney.
    D. Right kidney.

26. Light friction, petrissage, and effleurage are strokes that:
    A. Stimulate.
    B. Sedate.
    C. Aggravate.
    D. Roll.

27. A mass of blood trapped in the tissue is known as:
    A. Hematoma.
    B. Edema.
    C. Laceration.
    D. Ischemia.

28. Massage strokes directed toward the heart are:
    A. Centripetal.
    B. Centrifugal.
    C. Deep.
    D. Always indicated.

29. When applying deep strokes, too much pressure will cause the muscle to:
    A. Relax.
    B. Jump.
    C. Cramp.
    D. Roll.

30. In cross-fiber friction, the direction of movement over the intended area is:
    A. Vertical.
    B. Horizontal.
    C. Ipsilateral.
    D. Transverse.

31. Massage reappeared during the:
    A. Renaissance.
    B. Middle Ages.
    C. Dark Ages.
    D. Revolution.

32. The MT should contact client physician for all of the following except:
    A. Osteoporosis.
    B. Cancer.
    C. Osteoarthritis.
    D. Complicated pregnancy.

33. In the side-lying position, a pillow/bolster should be placed between the knees and under the:
    A. Head.
    B. Ankles.
    C. Shoulder.
    D. Leg.

34. A floating blood clot is known as a(n):
    A. Edema.
    B. Embolus.
    C. Thrombus.
    D. Infection.

35. Massaging a client with medication controlled hypertension should be:
    A. Soothing.
    B. Stimulating.
    C. Brisk.
    D. Not done.

36. Caution is used to avoid injuring underlying anatomical structures in:
    A. Contraindications.
    B. Cancer.
    C. Pneumonia.
    D. Endangerment areas.

37. Which oil is not used in massage because it can clog pores?
    A. Olive.
    B. Mineral.
    C. Rosewood.
    D. Jojoba.

38. Proteins that immunize the body are:
    A. Pathogens.
    B. Antigens.
    C. Antibodies.
    D. Endocrines.

39. The most important procedure in deterring the spread of germs by the MT is:
    A. Wearing short nails.
    B. Wearing scrubs.
    C. Using aromatherapy.
    D. Hand-washing.

40. The intake procedure before a massage includes all of the following except:
    A. Height of client.
    B. Medical history check list.
    C. Client observation.
    D. Verbal questioning.

41. Effleurage can be performed using all of the following except:
    A. Hands.
    B. Fingers.
    C. Toes.
    D. Arms.

42. Which stroke is used to reduce adhesions, separate muscle fibers, promote hyperemia and milk the tissue of metabolic wastes?
    A. Effleurage.
    B. Petrissage.

    C. Friction.
    D. Vibration.

43. Active assistive joint movement requires:
    A. Client only moving the extremity.
    B. Therapist only moving the extremity.
    C. Client and therapist moving the extremity together.
    D. The joint to be immobilized.

44. An MT is required to keep all client information:
    A. On public record.
    B. Confidential.
    C. In charts.
    D. At the MT's lawyer's office.

45. A treatment protocol using passive positioning is:
    A. Polarity.
    B. Strain-counterstrain.
    C. MET.
    D. CRAC.

46. This stroke creates the most heat in the tissue:
    A. Effleurage.
    B. Petrissage.
    C. Friction.
    D. Vibration.

47. The following is contraindicated for massage:
    A. Obesity.
    B. Osteoarthritis.
    C. Sunburn.
    D. Edema.

48. The most effective hydrotherapy treatment of sub-acute injuries is:
    A. Paraffin only.
    B. Heat only.
    C. Cryotherapy only.
    D. Contrast application of heat and cold.

49. Dr. Janet Travell was the founder of:
    A. Trigger point therapy.   C. Hellerwork.
    B. Rolfing.   D. Shiatsu.

50. Paraffin should never be applied over the:
    A. Wrist.
    B. Spine.
    C. Heart.
    D. Toes.

51. Water temperatures above or below the body temperature will have this effect when applied:
    A. Chemical.
    B. Thermal.
    C. Mechanical.
    D. Tertiary.

52. All of the following are contraindications for hydrotherapy except:
    A. Cardiac conditions.
    B. Diabetes.
    C. Kidney disease.
    D. Sub-acute sprain.

53. Bone reabsorption happens through the activity of the:
    A. Osteoblasts.
    B. Osteoclasts.
    C. Osteocytes.
    D. Osteotriocytes.

54. The cells responsible for transport of oxygen/carbon dioxide are:
    A. Leukocytes.
    B. Adipocytes.
    C. Osteocytes.
    D. Erythrocytes.

55. The period between initial stimulation and contraction is the:
    A. Latent.
    B. Refractory.
    C. Relaxation.
    D. Contractile.

56. The plantarflexor that crosses both the knee and ankle is the:
    A. Soleus.
    B. Gastrocnemius.
    C. Peroneus brevis.
    D. Tibialis posterior.

57. The origin of the rectus femoris is:
    A. ASIS.
    B. SIIS.
    C. AIIS.
    D. PSIS.

58. The function of insulin is to:
    A. Lower blood glucose levels.
    B. Rise blood glucose levels.
    C. Raise blood pressure.
    D. Lower blood pressure.

59. Another name for the pacemaker is the:
    A. AV node.
    B. SA node.
    C. Mitral valve.
    D. Tricuspid valve.

60. The molecule which binds oxygen and carbon dioxide in erythrocytes is:
    A. Thrombin.
    B. Thermogin.
    C. Hemoglobin.
    D. Antigen.

61. Coordination and balance are controlled by the:
    A. Cerebrum.
    B. Cerebellum.
    C. Pituitary.
    D. Thyroid.

62. The basic structural and functional unit of all living things is:
    A. Fibroblast.
    B. Molecule.
    C. Cell.
    D. Tissue.

63. The "master gland" is:
    A. Thyroid.
    B. Parathyroid.
    C. Pineal.
    D. Pituitary.

64. This plane divides the body into equal right and left halves:
    A. Mid-sagittal.
    B. Coronal.
    C. Sagittal.
    D. Frontal.

65. A client complains of pain in both hips. The proper nomenclature for the pain would be:
    A. Contralateral.
    B. Ipsilateral.
    C. Bilateral.
    D. Unilateral.

66. The body cavity which contains the thoracic and abdominopelvic regions is:
    A. Dorsal.
    B. Ventral.
    C. Vertebral.
    D. Cranial.

67. This muscle separates the thoracic and abdominopelvic regions:
    A. Esophagus.
    B. Rectus abdominis.
    C. Diaphragm.
    D. Serratus anterior.

68. Glands are made up of:
    A. Epitral tissue.
    B. Nervous tissue.
    C. Connective tissue.
    D. Epithelial tissue.

69. The nerve entrapped in carpal tunnel syndrome:
    A. Radial.
    B. Median.
    C. Ulnar.
    D. Femoral.

70. These muscles are known as entrappers because they can entrap a nerve or nerve plexus:
    A. Brachioradialis, biceps, scalenes.
    B. Scalenes, piriformis, pectoralis minor.
    C. Biceps, piriformis, scalenes.
    D. Pectoralis minor, biceps, brachioradialis.

71. Which muscle inserts on the styloid process of the radius?
    A. Brachioradialis
    B. Biceps brachii
    C. Brachialis
    D. Triceps long head

72. The gallbladder function is to:
    A. Store bile.
    B. Store insulin.
    C. Create insulin.
    D. Create meninges.

73. The outermost layer of the spinal cord is called:
    A. Pia mater.
    B. Arachnoid.
    C. Dura mater.
    D. Plexus.

74. Inflammation of any peripheral nerve is called:
    A. Nephritis.
    B. Neuritis.
    C. Neuronitis.
    D. Neurotonitis.

75. The reflex monitoring the length of a muscle spindle is called:
    A. Tendon reflex.
    B. Ipsilateral reflex.
    C. Stretch reflex.
    D. Sciatica.

76. Contraction of the serratus anterior will cause scapular:
    A. Protraction.
    B. Retraction.
    C. Elevation
    D. Depression.

77. How many types of tissue are there?
    A. 3
    B. 5
    C. 4
    D. 2

78. The function of epithelial tissue is:
    A. Protection, filtration, secretion.
    B. Binding, secretion, filtration.
    C. Connecting, protection, secretion.
    D. Building, filtration, connection.

79. The most abundant tissue in the body:
    A. Nervous.
    B. Muscle.
    C. Epithelial.
    D. Connective.

80. This neuron carries impulses toward the CNS:
    A. Efferent.
    B. Afferent.
    C. Myelin.
    D. Associative.

81. Protein synthesis occurs in the:
    A. Ribosome.
    B. Nucleus.
    C. Mitochondria.
    D. Golgi apparatus.

82. Proteins are composed of:
    A. Carbohydrates.
    B. Lipids.
    C. Amino acids.
    D. Nucleic acids.

83. Which of the following is not considered a formed element?
    A. Erythrocyte
    B. Plasma
    C. Leukocyte
    D. Thrombocyte

84. All of the following laterally rotate the humerus except:
    A. Infraspinatus.
    B. Teres minor.
    C. Deltoid.
    D. Teres major.

85. The epithelial layer of skin is known as:
    A. Epidermis.
    B. Dermis.

C. Subcutaneous.
D. Connective.

86. Pruritis means:
    A. Fungus.
    B. Bacteria.
    C. Pain.
    D. Itching.

87. Contraction of the semitendinosus will cause the knee to:
    A. Extend.
    B. Flex.
    C. Laterally rotate
    D. Circumduct.

88. During a massage, your client gets a cramp in the hamstrings. What should you do?
    A. Flex the knee and have your client contract the hamstrings
    B. Straighten the knee and have your client contract the quadriceps
    C. Flex the knee and have your client contract the tibialis anterior
    D. Straighten the knee and have your client flex the tibialis posterior

89. The medial leg bone is:
    A. Femur.
    B. Fibula.
    C. Tibia.
    D. Calcaneus.

90. Contraction of the teres major muscle will cause the teres minor to become:
    A. Shortened.
    B. Lengthened.
    C. Spasmodic.
    D. Cramping.

91. An antagonist to the tibialis anterior is:
    A. Extensor digitorum longus.
    B. Extensor hallucis longus.
    C. Peroneus tertius.
    D. Soleus.

92. A synergist to the gluteus medius in abduction of the hip is:
    A. Gracilis.
    B. Pectineus.
    C. Tensor fascia latae.
    D. Adductor magnus.

93. Contraction of the iliopsoas will cause the pectineus to:
    A. Lengthen.
    B. Shorten.
    C. Spasm.
    D. Cramp.

94. Engaging this muscle will bring the arm forward:
    A. Latissimus dorsi.
    B. Teres major.
    C. Infraspinatus.
    D. Coracobrachialis.

95. This muscle is used when rising from a seated position:
    A. Gluteus maximus.
    B. Gluteus medius.
    C. Gluteus minimus.
    D. Tensor fascia latae.

96. External rotation of the humerus will cause the palm of the hand to:
    A. Retract.
    B. Protract.
    C. Supinate.
    D. Pronate.

97. The most important step in CPR is:
    A. Calling 911.
    B. Opening the airway.
    C. Breathing.
    D. Checking for a pulse.

98. The first and foremost rule of massage is:
    A. Refer when necessary.
    B. Get fees up front.
    C. Do no harm.
    D. Truth in advertising.

99. A client reports having pain across the middle of her back. Which muscle may be involved?
    A. Quadratus lumborum
    B. Supraspinatus
    C. Teres minor
    D. Rhomboids

100. An antagonist to the biceps is the:
    A. Pronator teres.
    B. Brachialis.
    C. Brachioradialis.
    D. Supinator.

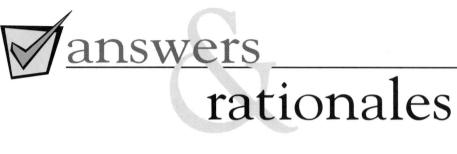

answers & rationales

The answer key will give you two pieces of information. The first is the correct answer, the second is the rationale.

1.
C. Both the tibialis anterior and posterior are involved in shin splints

2.
A. Yin energy flows inferior to superior

3.
D. Review the referral patterns in the text

4.
A. In polarity, gunas are the three types of touch

5.
B. Review the information in the text

6.
C. Post-event massage is to release toxin build-up and increase the amount of parasympathetic activity

7.
A. Displacement of the vertebrae may be caused by an imbalance in the spinal muscle contractions

8.
D. Review the referral patterns in the text

9.
B. With terminally ill patients, the therapist should offer relaxation massage

10.
A. Tsubos refers to Eastern Therapies.

11.
A. The therapist should work to make the mother as comfortable as possible

12.
C. All other yang meridians are on the back or lateral aspect of the body

13.
B. Sympathetic is fight-or-flight response

14.
D. The somatic (soma—body) nervous system is part of the PNS

15.
D. Key word: abdomen

16.
A. The only meridian that starts on the plantar surface of the foot

17.
C. The deepest stroke in massage

18.
D. The client does not assist, therefore eliminating muscular or tendinous involvement

19.
A. Where all power comes from

20.
B. The triceps extend the humerus

21.
D. Never proceed on an injury you or the client are unsure of

22.
A. Friction breaks down adhesions and scar tissue

23.
B. Type I diabetes—deficiency in insulin

24.
C. Hyperemia—influx of blood to an area

25.
B. Remember: The tricuspid (tri—three) valve is in the right side of the heart and there are three lobes in the right lung

26.
B. Heavy percussion/vibration stimulate

27.
A. Medical term meaning bruise

28.
A. Centrifugal—away from

29.
C. The spindle cell mechanism thinks the muscle is overstretched

30.
D. Cross-fiber—across the muscle fiber

31.
A. Massage disappeared during the Middle Ages

32.
C. Osteoarthritis is arthritis

33.
A. The therapist should work to make the client as comfortable as possible

34.
B. Thrombus—a stationary clot

35.
A. Key words: medication-controlled

36.
D. Contraindication—treatment is inadvisable

37.
B. Natural vegetable oils are fine for massage

38.
C. Key word: immunize

39.
D. The single most important way to protect yourself and your client

40.
A. This choice is the least important

41.
C. Most laws do not include the use of toes

42.
B. Key words: milks the tissue

43.
C. Client only—active; therapist only—passive

44.
B. Not only the law, but good ethics and professionalism

45.
B. Polarity—energy; CRAC is a form of MET

46.
C. The deepest stroke, therefore creates the most heat

47.
C. Particularly if there are blisters

48.
D. Contrast therapy has been proven to be most effective on chronic injuries

49.
A. Review adjunct therapy section in text

50.
C. Never over the heart or artificial joints

51.
B. Anything having to do with temperature is thermal

52.
D. Hydrotherapy is a recommended treatment for sub-acute injuries

53.
B. Osteoblasts and osteocytes build bone

54.
D. Erythrocytes—red blood cells

55.
A. Contractile period is when the muscle contracts

56.
B. The soleus only crosses the ankle joint

57.
C. Anterior inferior iliac spine

58.
A. Glucagon increases blood glucose levels

59.
B. Sinoatrial node

60.
C. Thrombin is involved in clotting

61.
B. Cerebrum—"the seat of intelligence"

62.
C. Molecules are made up of atoms; tissues are made up of cells

63.
D. Review endocrine system in text

64.
A. Sagittal divides the body into unequal right and left segments

65.
C. Contralateral—opposite; ipsilateral—same side; unilateral—one side

66.
B. Dorsal—cranial and spinal cavities

67.
C. Thorax—chest; abdominopelvic—abdomen and pelvis

68.
D. Epithelial tissue lines and protects the viscera

69.
B. The flexor tendons and retinaculum compress on the median nerve

70.
B. Scalenes—brachial plexus; pectoralis minor—axillary nerve; piriformis—sciatic nerve

71.
A. Named for its origin and insertion

72.
A. The pancreas is involved with insulin

73.
C. Dura mater translated, literally means "tough mother"

74.
B. Nephritis—inflammation of the nephron

75.
C. Tendon reflex is monitored by the Golgi tendon apparatus

76.
A. The strongest protractor of the scapula

77.
C. Review tissues in text

78.
A. Protection, filtration, and secretion to and from the outside of the body

79.
D. Surrounds and connects everything in the body

80.
B. Efferent nerves carry impulses away from the CNS

81.
A. Mitochondria—power house; Golgi apparatus—transports proteins; nucleus—controls all cell activity

82.
C. Nucleic acids make up DNA

83.
B. Plasma is what is left of the blood after the formed elements are removed

84.
D. Teres major medially rotates the humerus; posterior deltoid laterally rotates the humerus; anterior and middle deltoid medially rotate

85.
A. Dermis is composed of connective tissue

86.
D. Review definition of the integumentary system in the text

87.
B. The hamstrings extend the hip and flex the knee

88.
B. Reciprocal inhibition

89.
C. Fibula—lateral

90.
B. When the humerus is medially rotated, the teres minor will stretch because its action is lateral rotation

91.
D. Soleus plantar—flexes the foot

92.
C. The other three choices adduct the hip

93.
B. The pectineus also flexes the hip

94.
D. The only muscle listed that is on the front of the body

95.
A. The "power muscle"

96.
C. External rotation is the same as lateral rotation

97.
A. You want to make sure advanced life support is on the way

98.
C. The universal rule of massage

99.
D. Key words: middle of the back

100.
A. The biceps and the supinator supinate the forearm

Index